Interventional Radiology

Editor

DANA L. CLARKE

VETERINARY CLINICS OF NORTH AMERICA: SMALL ANIMAL PRACTICE

www.vetsmall.theclinics.com

September 2018 • Volume 48 • Number 5

ELSEVIER

1600 John F. Kennedy Boulevard • Suite 1800 • Philadelphia, Pennsylvania, 19103-2899
http://www.vetsmall.theclinics.com

VETERINARY CLINICS OF NORTH AMERICA: SMALL ANIMAL PRACTICE Volume 48, Number 5
September 2018 ISSN 0195-5616, ISBN-13: 978-0-323-64318-4

Editor: Colleen Dietzler
Developmental Editor: Meredith Madeira

Veterinary Clinics of North America: Small Animal Practice (ISSN 0195-5616) is published bimonthly by Elsevier Inc., 360 Park Avenue South, New York, NY 10010-1710. Months of issue are January, March, May, July, September, and November. Business and Editorial Offices: 1600 John F. Kennedy Blvd., Ste. 1800, Philadelphia, PA 19103-2899. Customer Service Office: 3251 Riverport Lane, Maryland Heights, MO 63043. Periodicals postage paid at New York, NY and additional mailing offices. Subscription prices are $325.00 per year (domestic individuals), $622.00 per year (domestic institutions), $100.00 per year (domestic students/residents), $430.00 per year (Canadian individuals), $773.00 per year (Canadian institutions), $469.00 per year (international individuals), $773.00 per year (international institutions), and $220.00 per year (international and Canadian students/residents). To receive student/resident rate, orders must be accompanied by name of affiliated institution, date of term, and the *signature* of program/residency coordinator on institution letterhead. Orders will be billed at individual rate until proof of status is received. Foreign air speed delivery is included in all *Clinics* subscription prices. All prices are subject to change without notice. **POSTMASTER:** Send address changes to *Veterinary Clinics of North America: Small Animal Practice*, Elsevier Health Sciences Division, Subscription Customer Service, 3251 Riverport Lane, Maryland Heights, MO 63043. Customer Service (orders, claims, online, change of address): Elsevier Periodicals Customer Service, Elsevier Health Sciences Division Subscription **Customer Service 3251 Riverport Lane Maryland Heights, MO 63043. Tel: 1-800-654-2452 (U.S. and Canada); 314-447-8871 (outside U.S. and Canada). Fax: 314-447-8029. E-mail: journalscustomerservice-usa@elsevier.com (for print support); journalsonlinesupport-usa@elsevier.com (for online support).**

Reprints. For copies of 100 or more of articles in this publication, please contact the Commercial Reprints Department, Elsevier Inc., 360 Park Avenue South, New York, NY 10010-1710. Tel.: 212-633-3874; Fax: 212-633-3820; E-mail: reprints@elsevier.com.

Veterinary Clinics of North America: Small Animal Practice is also published in Japanese by Inter Zoo Publishing Co., Ltd., Aoyama Crystal-Bldg 5F, 3-5-12 Kitaaoyama, Minato-ku, Tokyo 107-0061, Japan.

Veterinary Clinics of North America: Small Animal Practice is covered in *Current Contents/Agriculture, Biology and Environmental Sciences, Science Citation Index, ASCA, MEDLINE/PubMed (Index Medicus), Excerpta Medica,* and *BIOSIS.*

Contributors

EDITOR

DANA L. CLARKE, VMD
Diplomate, American College of Veterinary Emergency and Critical Care; Assistant Professor of Interventional Radiology and Critical Care, Department of Clinical Sciences and Advanced Medicine, University of Pennsylvania School of Veterinary Medicine, Philadelphia, Pennsylvania, USA

AUTHORS

MATTHEW W. BEAL, DVM
Diplomate, American College of Veterinary Emergency and Critical Care; Professor, Emergency and Critical Care Medicine and Interventional Radiology, Department of Small Animal Clinical Sciences, Michigan State University, East Lansing, Michigan, USA

DANA L. CLARKE, VMD
Diplomate, American College of Veterinary Emergency and Critical Care; Assistant Professor of Interventional Radiology and Critical Care, Department of Clinical Sciences and Advanced Medicine, University of Pennsylvania, School of Veterinary Medicine, Philadelphia, Pennsylvania, USA

ANDRÉANNE CLÉROUX, DMV
Diplomate, American College of Veterinary Internal Medicine (Small Animal Internal Medicine); Lecturer in Internal Medicine and Interventional Radiology, Department of Clinical Studies, University of Pennsylvania, School of Veterinary Medicine, Philadelphia, Pennsylvania, USA

WILLIAM T.N. CULP, VMD
Diplomate, American College of Veterinary Surgeons; ACVS Founding Fellow of Minimally Invasive Surgery, ACVS Founding Fellow of Surgical Oncology, Associate Professor, Department of Surgical and Radiological Sciences, School of Veterinary Medicine, University of California, Davis, Davis, California, USA

MARILYN DUNN, DVM, MVSc
Diplomate, American College of Veterinary Internal Medicine (Small Animal Internal Medicine); Professor, Interventional Radiology and Endoscopy, CHUV Faculty of Veterinary Medicine, University of Montreal, Quebec, Canada

ALEXANDER GALLAGHER, DVM, MS
Diplomate, American College of Veterinary Internal Medicine (Small Animal Internal Medicine); Clinical Assistant Professor, Small Animal Medicine, Department of Small Animal Clinical Sciences, College of Veterinary Medicine, University of Florida, Gainesville, Florida, USA

MAUREEN A. GRIFFIN, DVM
Department of Surgical and Radiological Sciences, School of Veterinary Medicine, University of California, Davis, Davis, California, USA

REBECCA HERSH-BOYLE, DVM
Department of Radiological and Surgical Sciences, University of California, Davis, School
of Veterinary Medicine, Davis, California

JEFFREY I. MONDSCHEIN, MD
Associate Professor of Clinical Radiology and Surgery, Attending Interventional Radiologist,
Department of Radiology, Perelman School of Medicine, University of Pennsylvania,
Hospital of the University of Pennsylvania, Philadelphia, Pennsylvania, USA

BRIAN A. SCANSEN, DVM, MS
Diplomate, American College of Veterinary Internal Medicine (Cardiology); Associate
Professor, Section Head, Cardiology and Cardiac Surgery, Department of Clinical
Sciences, Colorado State University, Fort Collins, Colorado, USA

Contents

> Interventional radiology is a subspecialty of diagnostic radiology that uses minimally invasive techniques performed under imaging guidance. Interventional radiology has its roots in angiography, which is the radiologic examination of blood vessels after the introduction of a contrast medium that allows them to be imaged. Going forward, the collaboration between human and veterinary interventional radiologists will persist as a two-way street and will continue to innovate together and learn from each other and from the patients.

> Interventional radiology in veterinary medicine was adapted from techniques developed in human medicine and has a variety of applications to treat disease in multiple body systems. Fluoroscopy is required for almost all interventional procedures, requiring knowledge of proper safety techniques for working with ionizing radiation. There are a wide variety of catheters, wires, sheaths, stents, and embolics used in veterinary medicine. Familiarity with their indications and sizing compatibility is essential for procedural success.

> Chondromalacia of the tracheal and bronchial cartilages and redundancy of the dorsal tracheal membrane result in collapse of the large airways, leading to coughing and airway obstruction. It most commonly affects small-breed dogs, although larger-breed dogs, cats, and miniature horses are also sporadically reported. Dynamic airway imaging is used to confirm the diagnosis. The primary goal of medical management is to control clinical signs attributable to coughing and airway inflammation. When this is no longer effective, tracheal stents provide a minimally invasive, rapid way to restore airway patency. Bronchial stenting is in its infancy in veterinary medicine.

> Vascular malformations are abnormal connections between blood vessels that can have various endothelial characteristics. Although uncommon, these malformations can present challenging diagnostic and therapeutic

scenarios. The use of interventional radiology techniques in the management of various vascular malformations is an attractive option because of the ability to treat these malformations at the most appropriate anatomic location and in the most effective manner. Techniques such as coil embolization of intrahepatic portosystemic shunts and liquid embolization of arteriovenous fistulae/malformations have shown tremendous potential as treatments for these challenging diseases.

Cardiac Interventions in Small Animals: Areas of Uncertainty

Brian A. Scansen

There remain areas of uncertainty in optimal technique, preferred candidates, and expected outcome for small animal patients undergoing cardiac intervention. This article highlights issues within interventional cardiology that are in need of study and offers the author's opinion and experience on topics such as variants of pulmonary valve anatomy and alternatives to conventional balloon dilation for pulmonary valve stenosis, patient selection for cutting or high-pressure balloon dilation of aortic valvar or subaortic stenosis, occlusion of patent ductus arteriosus in very small dogs, ductal stenting in conditions with reduced pulmonary blood flow, and alternative considerations for vascular access and closure.

Interventional Radiology Management of Vascular Obstruction

Marilyn Dunn and Brian A. Scansen

Vascular obstructions in small animals have numerous causes and variable signs depending on location and chronicity. The decision to treat and by which method (medical, interventional, surgical) can be challenging. A combined approach of catheter-directed thrombolysis, angioplasty, or vascular stenting may be most appropriate for acute thrombosis, although optimal therapeutic strategies are undefined in this population. The role of embolic trapping devices in animals is uncertain. Chronic cases of vascular obstruction, with collateral flow and neither ischemia nor venous congestion manifest, may be conservatively managed. Prospective clinical studies are needed to better guide management of vascular obstructions in veterinary medicine.

Interventional Radiology and Interventional Endoscopy in Treatment of Nephroureteral Disease in the Dog and Cat

Alexander Gallagher

Interventional endoscopy and interventional radiology have led to the development of minimally invasive techniques for management of kidney and ureteral diseases in the dog and cat, including idiopathic renal hematuria, ureteral obstruction, and ectopic ureters. Sclerotherapy is a renal-sparing chemical cauterization technique used in cases of idiopathic renal hematuria. Diagnosis of ureteral obstruction is challenging in some cases based on ultrasound imaging alone, and antegrade pyelography should be considered. Treatment options for obstructions include nephrostomy tubes, ureteral stents, and subcutaneous ureteral bypass devices. Treatment with cystoscopic-guided laser ablation provides similar outcomes to surgery in dogs with intramural ectopic ureters.

Matthew W. Beal

> Lower urinary tract (LUT) emergencies are common reasons for small animal patients to be presented to their veterinarians. Patient stabilization and management of life-threatening problems is a priority in this population. Urethral obstruction is a common LUT emergency. Urethral stent placement has gained popularity over the past decade, allowing for a minimally invasive, image-guided method for relief of urethral obstruction in some patient populations. This article focuses on candidate selection, diagnostic workup, stent placement technique, and the expected outcome and complications for patients undergoing urethral stent placement and addresses some additional strategies for interventional management of LUT emergencies.

Andréanne Cléroux

> Urolithiasis commonly affects cats and dogs. The American College of Veterinary Internal Medicine established guidelines for the treatment of uroliths that reflect modern techniques prioritizing minimally invasive procedures, with an emphasis on prevention strategies to limit morbidity and mortality. Extracorporeal shockwave lithotripsy and endoscopic nephrolithotomy constitute some of the minimally invasive treatment modalities available for upper urinary tract uroliths. Cystoscopic-guided basket retrieval, cystoscopic-guided laser lithotripsy, and percutaneous cystolithotomy are minimally invasive options for the management of lower urinary tract uroliths. Following stone removal, prevention strategies are essential to help reduce morbidity and mortality associated with stone recurrence.

William T.N. Culp

> Whenever possible, surgical removal of tumors should be pursued because this likely allows for the best possible outcome for a particular patient; however, this may not be pursued for various reasons. In those situations, interventional radiology (IR) options can be considered as definitive therapy or palliation. Locoregional therapies such as intraarterial chemotherapy and embolization/chemoembolization, although rarely reported in veterinary medicine, offer an alternative minimally invasive treatment option. In addition, drainage of body fluids or neoplastic effusions can be established via IR means, and when tumors are not removed but luminal patency needs to be reestablished, palliative stenting can also be performed.

VETERINARY CLINICS OF NORTH AMERICA: SMALL ANIMAL PRACTICE

Preface

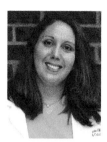

Dana L. Clarke, VMD
Editor

Over the last 25 years, there has been a surge in the availability and expertise in minimally invasive procedures in veterinary medicine. As we have continued to push technique, equipment, and case selection boundaries, veterinary Interventional Radiology (IR) has evolved from procedures previously performed solely by veterinary cardiologists and radiologists to an exciting, promising subspecialty in veterinary medicine with applications for all body systems.

Veterinary IR is still in its infancy compared with IR in human medicine. Human IR has rapidly expanded in both physician numbers and breadth of capabilities since the description of needle- and wire-guided vascular access in 1952 by Dr Sven Ivar Seldinger and the first arterial angioplasty performed by Dr Charles Dotter in 1963. Veterinary IR emerged from a close relationship with human IR at one of the largest IR human programs at the Hospital of the University of Pennsylvania in the late 1990s. Many veterinarians performing IR today routinely consult with their human counterparts for advice and case assistance given our overall limited experience compared with physicians specialized in IR. Given veterinary IR's translational roots, the potential for solving human and veterinary health issues through collaboration, creativity, and inventiveness has yet to be fully realized.

Veterinary IR is uniquely positioned for innovative growth since there is no set career path to becoming a veterinary interventionalist; we are surgeons, internists, criticalists, cardiologists, and radiologists. Through our advanced training, we bring our proficiency and expertise to a multidisciplinary specialty that requires incorporation of all aspects of medicine for successful patient outcomes. We contribute our perspective, talents, and knowledge to create a subspecialty that truly blends the best of veterinary medicine.

This issue of *Veterinary Clinics of North America: Small Animal Practice* outlines the fascinating history of IR in human medicine and how procedures designed to address human diseases through image-guided techniques have been adapted for our veterinary patients. It also details common conditions that can be addressed by IR, including some that are still considered investigational, particularly within the realm of managing

Vet Clin Small Anim 48 (2018) ix–x
https://doi.org/10.1016/j.cvsm.2018.06.001
0195-5616/18/© 2018 Published by Elsevier Inc.

vascular obstructions. The article on cardiology challenges what we know and how we approach minimally invasive cardiac procedures, and the article on interventional management of nonresectable neoplasia sheds light on what will likely be one of the fastest growing applications of IR in veterinary medicine: interventional oncology. The authors in this issue are actively developing the field of veterinary IR, and I appreciate their time and effort invested for our collective veterinary IR knowledge expansion.

The future is bright for veterinary IR. Our unique skill sets stemming from varied specialty backgrounds and love of a challenge will be what attracts the best and brightest to this field, ensuring it becomes a successful stand-alone specialty in veterinary medicine. It has been a privilege to edit this issue, and I sincerely thank the team of talented, dedicated veterinarian authors who not only contributed articles but also work tirelessly toward the scientific advancement IR in veterinary medicine.

With my most sincere thanks,

Dana L. Clarke, VMD
Department of Clinical Sciences and
Advanced Medicine
University of Pennsylvania School of Veterinary Medicine
Philadelphia, PA 19104, USA

E-mail address:
clarked@vet.upenn.edu

Perspectives from Human Interventional Radiology

Jeffrey I. Mondschein, MD

KEYWORDS

- Interventional radiology • Radiograph • Stenosis • X-ray imaging

KEY POINTS

- Interventional radiology is a subspecialty of diagnostic radiology that uses minimally invasive techniques performed under imaging guidance.
- Numerous medical scientists and physician-scientists have played important roles in the advancement of human interventional radiology, and their discoveries and thought processes served as the foundations for innovative procedures that subsequently developed within veterinary medicine.
- Image-guided minimally invasive procedures have been used to treat myriad conditions and solve innumerable therapeutic puzzles for human patients since the 1960s, but the field nonetheless continues to evolve and adapt at an incredible pace.
- Going forward, the collaboration between human and veterinary interventional radiologists will persist as a two-way street, and we will continue to innovate together and learn from each other and from our patients.

Interventional radiology is a subspecialty of diagnostic radiology that uses minimally invasive techniques performed under imaging guidance. Although it is sometimes referred to as image-guided surgery, most procedures performed by interventional radiologists use skin incisions that are less than 5 mm in length. In human patients, most of the procedures are performed using local anesthetic only or local anesthesia combined with moderate sedation. General anesthesia is rarely necessary. Recovery time from these procedures is typically short, and up to 80% can be performed on an outpatient basis, with patients going home the same day.

Interventional radiology has its roots in angiography, which is the radiologic examination of blood vessels after the introduction of a contrast medium that allows them to be imaged. The first angiogram was performed only months after radiographs were discovered by German physicist Wilhelm Roentgen in 1895. Two physicians in Vienna injected mercury salts into an amputated hand from a cadaver and created an image of the arteries in January, 1896. Egas Moniz, a Portuguese physician, developed the technique for use in living human subjects and performed the first cerebral angiogram

Department of Radiology, Perelman School of Medicine at the University of Pennsylvania, Hospital of the University of Pennsylvania, 3400 Spruce Street, 1 Silverstein Building, Philadelphia, PA 19104, USA
E-mail address: Jeffrey.Mondschein@uphs.upenn.edu

Vet Clin Small Anim 48 (2018) 743–749
https://doi.org/10.1016/j.cvsm.2018.05.001
0195-5616/18/© 2018 Elsevier Inc. All rights reserved.
vetsmall.theclinics.com

in 1927. By the 1930s, angiography became the first interventional radiology procedure performed in human subjects for diagnostic purposes.[1]

In 1953, Dr Sven Ivar Seldinger described a technique that enhanced the safety of angiography. Before his work, large bore needles were used to access arteries, and liquid radiopaque contrast was either injected directly for x-ray imaging or a smaller catheter was placed via the needle into the blood vessel and used for the contrast injection. Because of the large size of the necessary instruments for this technique, it could only be used to access large diameter blood vessels such as the aorta. Also, because it created a large hole in the artery on removal of the instruments, hemorrhage and arterial wall injury were frequent complications. Seldinger refined the procedure by placing a flexible guidewire through the needle after vascular access. The needle was removed, leaving the guidewire behind as a placeholder that bridged the space between the skin surface and the blood vessel lumen. Then, a thin-walled, flexible plastic catheter was threaded over the wire and placed percutaneously into the blood vessel.[2]

Seldinger's method was a very important enhancement in radiologic technique, because it allowed a catheter of similar diameter to the original access needle to be inserted through the skin to the vessel below, obviating the need for a large bore needle or surgical exposure of the vessel. Smaller vessels could be used, including ones that were more superficial than the aorta. In the 1960s, femoral access became popular, because the femoral artery was superficial, palpable, and located anterior to the femoral head, which allowed for manual compression to achieve hemostasis following removal of the catheter. This technique ultimately allowed the field of interventional radiology to take root and grow. It was found to be useful not only for accessing blood vessels but also, in subsequent years, for obtaining percutaneous access to a variety of anatomic structures, including bile ducts, urinary collecting systems, stomach and bowel, lymphatics, and others.

Not long after Seldinger developed his technique, Charles T. Dotter became the chairman of the department of radiology at the University of Oregon. He was only 32 years of age when he took this post, and it was a position he held for over 30 years. He was known for being a brilliant innovator with tireless energy and an outspoken, flamboyant, and animated style. He is generally regarded as the father of interventional radiology. He invented several important devices, including Teflon catheters and flexible guidewires, and also developed rapid sequence film technology that allowed for improved diagnostic evaluation of arteries. Dotter was the first to perform percutaneous transluminal angioplasty to treat stenosis of an artery and published a paper describing the technique in 1964.[3] Of interest, the original angioplasty procedures that he performed did not make use of angioplasty balloons, which had not yet been invented for percutaneous use, but instead used multiple dilators of progressively larger size, placed over a guidewire and through the stenotic area to stretch it open. He subsequently went on to introduce arterial stenting and stent graft placement, as well as thrombolysis to dissolve blood clots using direct injection of streptokinase into the thrombus occluding the vessel. He also helped develop the loop snare, used to retrieve intravascular foreign bodies.[4]

In 1974, Andreas Gruntzig, a cardiologist in Switzerland, invented a balloon catheter for dilating vascular stenosis.[5] Melvin Judkins developed preshaped catheters that readily allow for coronary artery catheterization. Although interventional radiologists were instrumental in creating many of the original techniques and devices used in coronary angiography and interventions, interventional cardiology eventually branched off from interventional radiology and became a subspecialty of cardiology.

Since the early 1970s, interventional radiology has developed at a rapid rate. Many disease processes that previously could only be treated using open surgery, and some that were deemed too risky for surgical treatment, were subsequently addressed using minimally invasive, percutaneous techniques under imaging guidance. Because imaging techniques expanded from fluoroscopy and rapid sequence film to include ultrasound and computed tomography, almost the entire human body became accessible for image-guided access and intervention, and both safety and efficacy of interventions improved. The attributes that made this specialty attractive compared with classical surgical techniques included decreased risk, faster and less painful recovery, shortened hospital stay, and often significantly decreased cost.

Numerous medical scientists and physician-scientists have played important roles in the advancement of interventional radiology, and it would be impossible to credit them all in an article of this size and scope. However, mention of a select few help to illustrate the diversity of interventions that have been developed and the disease processes they can address.

Dr Josef Rosch, an interventional radiologist who served as the director of the Dotter Interventional Institute in Oregon, developed the transjugular intrahepatic portosystemic shunt (TIPS) procedure for the treatment of portal hypertension. This procedure allows for creation of an artificial conduit between the portal vein and a hepatic vein using a jugular venous approach and minimally invasive techniques under fluoroscopic guidance. Others subsequently refined the procedure, but before this innovation, portosystemic shunts could only be created surgically. Unfortunately, the patient population in need of this type of shunting is considered high risk for open surgery due to the potential for liver failure and mortality. Therefore, the minimally invasive option was considered a giant step in mitigating risk and expanding the number of patients who could benefit from treatment of portal hypertension. Today, TIPS procedures are frequently performed routinely. At the conclusion of the procedure, neck access incisions are so small that they do not require sutures and the patient will leave the interventional radiology procedure room with just a small covering adhesive bandage. Most patients will be monitored overnight and can go home from the hospital the following day.[6] Dr Rosch also described the technique of embolization for treatment of gastrointestinal bleeding.

Although angioplasty to treat arterial stenosis became a popular treatment, especially for coronary arteries, restenosis at the sites of prior angioplasty was a frequent issue. Julio Palmaz is an interventional radiologist who developed a balloon expandable stent that served as a scaffolding to hold the blood vessel open at the former site of stenosis by literally pushing atherosclerotic plaque aside. The stent consisted of a metal tube that had holes cut in it to make it collapsible. The stent could then be crimped onto a balloon catheter, giving it a very small diameter as it was being delivered. After balloon expansion at the desired site, the stent would expand to a larger diameter and would remain rigid even after the balloon was deflated.[7] Food and Drug Administration approval was achieved in 1991 for peripheral arteries and in 1994 for coronary arteries. Within 4 years, it was being used in most of the percutaneous coronary interventions. In the August 2002 issue, Intellectual Property Worldwide magazine heralded it as one of "Ten Patents that Changed the World" during the past century. Dr Palmaz also worked on early versions of stent grafts.

Constantin Cope was an interventional radiologist at the University of Pennsylvania who developed a variety of techniques and devices. His micropuncture set consists of a 21-guage needle with a very small caliber wire and catheter/dilator set, which allowed for very small diameter vascular access that would help limit the risk of vascular injury and hemorrhage. He also invented the locking Cope loop catheter.

Using percutaneous techniques, it is possible to place drainage catheters into fluid collections such as abscesses or in fluid-filled structures in organs like the renal collecting system and bile ducts that may require external drainage for decompression. However, the available drains were based on preexisting surgical drains that were basically straight, hollow tubes. Dr Cope was increasingly frustrated by the fact that these tubes had the tendency to back out over time and become malpositioned, because there was nothing to retain them internally. Externally, the catheter could readily slip through the external skin suture intended to secure the catheter. The Cope locking loop is a catheter that can be placed percutaneously to allow for fluid drainage and has a string that runs through the lumen and attaches to the catheter tip. After placement, the interventional radiologist pulls the string, which deflects the tip of the catheter within the fluid collection, forming a loop that helps prevent the catheter from being pulled out of the fluid cavity.[8] Toward the end of a career that included a wide range of innovations, Dr Cope pioneered the technique of thoracic duct embolization via percutaneous lymphatic system access in order to treat chyle leaks resulting in chylothorax and chylous ascites, conditions that were traditionally very difficult to successfully address surgically.

Sidney Wallace was an interventional radiologist who spent the large majority of his career at MD Anderson Cancer Center in Houston, Texas. He helped lay the groundwork for the development of arterial tumor embolization, especially in renal tumors, to be used preoperatively to limit intraoperative hemorrhage or as a stand-alone palliative therapy. His work also provided the basis for much of what has become the modern subspecialty of interventional oncology, which includes therapies such as transarterial chemoembolization (TACE), transarterial radioembolization (TARE), percutaneous biopsy, direct intratumoral injection of drugs, as well as thermal tumor ablation using radiofrequency, microwave energy, and cryoablation.

Interventional radiologists of today are involved in treating a wide variety of disease entities throughout the human body and are therefore involved in almost all medical disciplines to varying degrees. What started with diagnostic angiography has now grown to include the procedures noted earlier, as well as many others, including biliary drainage and stone removal, urinary drainage and stenting to relieve obstruction, abscess drainage, dialysis access maintenance, stroke interventions, embolization of vascular malformations, inferior vena cava filter placement for prevention of pulmonary embolism, placement of all types of venous access devices, uterine artery embolization to treat menorrhagia and bulk symptoms from uterine fibroids, varicocele embolization to treat male infertility, venous thrombectomy and stenting, enteral access and catheter placement for feeding and decompression, vertebroplasty and kyphoplasty for vertebral fractures, and percutaneous nerve blocks for pain. More recent developments with evolving roles include prostate artery embolization to treat benign prostatic hypertrophy, left gastric artery embolization to treat obesity, and geniculate artery embolization for osteoarthritis-related knee pain.

Large-scale collaboration between interventional radiologists and veterinarians blossomed more than 15 years ago. In the early days, a friendship developed between Jeffrey Solomon, MD, a self-proclaimed dog lover and interventional radiologist at the University of Pennsylvania, and Chick Weisse, VMD, DACVS, a veterinarian and small animal surgeon at the Veterinary Hospital of the University of Pennsylvania. Dr Weisse was completing his veterinary training at that time and subsequently went on to complete a customized fellowship in interventional radiology that included work at both the human and veterinary hospitals of the University of Pennsylvania.

This friendship ultimately developed into an innovative collaborative relationship that adapted techniques used in human interventional radiology to treat various pathologic processes in animals. Earlier in this article, it was noted that TIPS are communications created between the portal veins and systemic veins to decrease the portal pressure in human patients with portal hypertension. Dogs and cats can sometimes present with the opposite problem—congenital shunts that are preexisting abnormal communications between the portal and systemic veins, present from birth. Therefore, in animals, instead of trying to create these communications, the goal is to partially or fully occlude them. Solomon and Weisse described a technique that combined stent placement and coil embolization for partial closure as well as another technique using a septal occluder device for complete closure of congenital intrahepatic portosystemic shunts.[9,10]

Embolization techniques commonly used in human medicine were also found to be very useful in veterinary patients. Solomon and Weisse described percutaneous transarterial embolization and chemoembolization for treatment of both benign and malignant tumors in animals. They used TACE to treat nonresectable hepatocellular carcinoma palliatively in dogs and particle embolization to treat benign, nonresectable liver tumors in dogs for symptomatic relief. One of the more interesting and unusual procedures that they reported was use of particles for embolization of the uterine arteries in a goat that was experiencing menorrhagia due to uterine fibroids.[11] For these procedures, knowledge of the appearance of human vascular anatomy and pathology helped them to determine the vascular supply to the tumors while performing arteriograms in the animals. Embolization of the animal arteries was performed using the same techniques as those used for treatment of human subjects.

Solomon and Weisse also demonstrated the utility of minimally invasive interventional procedures to treat epistaxis in dogs (embolization), malignant bowel obstruction in cats (enteric stent placement), malignant urinary obstruction in dogs (ureteral and urethral stent placement), and tracheal stenosis or collapse in dogs and cats (tracheal stenting). They even made use of snares to retrieve intravascular foreign bodies from dogs, horses, and a goat. All of the above-mentioned procedures are commonly performed in humans for the same types of pathology. Given the similarities between humans and other mammals in anatomy, organ systems, and pathology, the ability to use minimally invasive tools and techniques from human medicine to treat animals is not surprising.[12–16]

On a personal note, the author remember these early collaborative days very well, because he assisted with the veterinary interventional procedures described earlier and continue to have an active role in the interventional radiology program at University of Pennsylvania School of Veterinary Medicine. It was a time of unprecedented excitement for the veterinarians because a new specialty was taking shape. For the interventional radiologists who until that time had only treated humans, it was also a renewal of faith in the healing power and problem-solving utility of minimally invasive, image-guided procedures. It is also a fact that interventional radiologists who practice human medicine, the author included, are frequently animal lovers as well, so helping to treat the animals has been a source of great satisfaction. The same advantages that are noted in human patients are also seen in animals—lower risk, less discomfort and quicker recovery, ability to treat lesions that may not be readily treated using operative techniques, and decreased length of hospital stay and need for intensive care unit care.

Decreased cost may ultimately be one of the most important arguments for the further development of veterinary interventional radiology. Although there is an initial high cost to obtain necessary imaging equipment and medical devices, these expenses can be made up in time. The real savings come from the shorter hospital stays and decreased complication rates compared with surgery. In a human patient population where medical insurance is common, these differences may not be as readily apparent to the patient and their family. However, in the veterinary population, insurance coverage is less common, and even when it does exist, it is frequently less comprehensive than the human counterpart. Therefore, it is hoped that the cost savings of interventional radiology may eventually increase access to health care for many animals and their owners.

It is now possible for a veterinarian to obtain formal training in interventional radiology at some veterinary academic programs, and veterinary interventional radiology services are being offered in multiple centers throughout the United States and around the world. Veterinarians already in practice are also attending courses to gain proficiency in the techniques. Device companies are beginning to create tools specifically designed for use in animals. Minimally invasive, image-guided veterinary treatments are becoming standard for a variety of the conditions previously mentioned. So although veterinary interventional radiology may be in its relative infancy compared with human interventional radiology, the field is growing at a rapid rate.

In summary, both human and veterinary interventional radiology have a very bright future. Image-guided minimally invasive procedures have been used to treat myriad conditions and solve innumerable therapeutic puzzles for human patients since the 1960s, but the field nonetheless continues to evolve and adapt at an incredible pace. Going forward, the collaboration between human and veterinary interventional radiologists will persist as a two-way street, and we will continue to innovate together and learn from each other and from our patients.

REFERENCES

1. Rösch J, Keller FS, Kaufman JA. The birth, early years, and future of interventional radiology. J Vasc Interv Radiol 2003;14(7):841–53.
2. Higgs ZC, Macafee DA, Braithwaite BD, et al. The Seldinger technique: 50 years on. Lancet 2005;366(9494):1407–9.
3. Dotter CT, Judkins MP. Transluminal treatment of arteriosclerotic obstruction.Description of a new technic and a preliminary report of its application. Circulation 1964;30:654–70.
4. Keller FS, Rosch J. A personal memoir of Charles Dotter [foreword]. In: The father of interventional radiology. Charles Dotter: highlights of his life and research. Tokyo: Excerpta Medica Publishers; 1994. p. 7–9.
5. Grüntzig AR, Senning A, Siegenthaler WE. Nonoperative dilatation of coronary-artery stenosis: percutaneous transluminal coronary angioplasty. N Engl J Med 1979;301(2):61–8.
6. Rösch J. Development of transjugular intrahepatic portosystemic shunt. J Vasc Interv Radiol 2015;26(2):220–2.
7. Palmaz JC, Sibbitt RR, Tio FO, et al. Expandable intraluminal vascular graft: a feasibility study. Surgery 1986;99(2):199–205.
8. Cope C. Improved anchoring of nephrostomy catheters: loop technique. AJR Am J Roentgenol 1980;135(2):402–3.
9. Weisse C, Schwartz K, Stronger R, et al. Transjugular coil embolization of an intrahepatic portosystemic shunt in a cat. J Am Vet Med Assoc 2002;221(9):1287–91, 1266–7.
10. Weisse C, Mondschein JI, Itkin M, et al. Use of a percutaneous atrial septaloccluder device for complete acute occlusion of an intrahepatic portosystemic shunt in a dog. J Am Vet Med Assoc 2005;227(2):249–52, 236.

11. Weisse C, Clifford CA, Holt D, et al. Percutaneous arterial embolization and che-moembolization for treatment of benign and malignant tumors in three dogs and a goat. J Am Vet Med Assoc 2002;221(10):1430–6, 1419.

12. Weisse C, Nicholson ME, Rollings C, et al. Use of percutaneous arterial emboli-zation for treatment of intractable epistaxis in three dogs. J Am Vet Med Assoc 2004;224(8):1307–11, 1281.

13. Hume DZ, Solomon JA, Weisse CW. Palliative use of a stent for colonic obstruc-tion caused by adenocarcinoma in two cats. J Am Vet Med Assoc 2006;228(3): 392–6.

14. Weisse C, Berent A, Todd K, et al. Evaluation of palliative stenting for manage-ment of malignant urethral obstructions in dogs. J Am Vet Med Assoc 2006; 229(2):226–34.

15. Culp WT, Weisse C, Cole SG, et al. Intraluminal tracheal stenting for treatment of tracheal narrowing in three cats. Vet Surg 2007;36(2):107–13.

16. Culp WT, Weisse C, Berent AC, et al. Percutaneous endovascular retrieval of an intravascular foreign body in five dogs, a goat, and a horse. J Am Vet Med Assoc 2008;232(12):1850–6.

Interventional Equipment and Radiation Safety

Andréanne Cléroux, DMV[a],*, Rebecca Hersh-Boyle, DVM[b],
Dana L. Clarke, VMD[c]

KEYWORDS

- Radiation • Fluoroscopy • Catheterization • Balloon dilation • Embolization • Stent
- Interventional radiology

KEY POINTS

- Veterinary interventional radiology was adapted from techniques developed in human medicine, and has a variety of applications to treat disease in multiple organ systems.
- Fluoroscopy is required for most interventional procedures, requiring knowledge of proper safety techniques for working with ionizing radiation.
- There are a wide variety of catheters, wires, sheaths, stents, and embolics used in veterinary medicine. Familiarity with their indications and sizing compatibility is essential for procedural success.

INTRODUCTION

Interventional radiology (IR) is a specialty that was first developed in human medicine and that uses minimally invasive image-guided techniques to allow the diagnosis and/ or treatment of a variety of conditions. In its infancy, it consisted only of diagnostic procedures, mainly angiography for cases such as neoplasia, gastrointestinal (GI) bleeding, deep vein thromboembolic disease, and vascular mapping before a surgical intervention.[1] Before the advent of IR, these procedures were only possible with the placement of catheters via surgical cutdowns.[2] In 1953, Dr. Sven Seldinger[3] described percutaneous vascular catheter placement following needle access, later named the Seldinger method, which laid the foundation for the development of IR. Shortly after, Dotter and Judkins,[4] using the Seldinger method to establish vascular access, described the transluminal treatment of arteriosclerotic obstructions using a guide and dilating catheters under fluoroscopic guidance, minimizing the limitations associated with the surgical correction of this condition, surgical trauma, and morbidity. This was a key step in

[a] Department of Clinical Sciences and Advanced Medicine, University of Pennsylvania, School of Veterinary Medicine, 3900 Spruce Street, Philadelphia, PA 19104, USA; [b] Department of Radiological and Surgical Sciences, University of California, Davis, School of Veterinary Medicine, 1 Shields Avenue, Davis, CA 95616, USA; [c] Department of Clinical Sciences and Advanced Medicine, University of Pennsylvania, Philadelphia, PA 19104, USA
* Corresponding author.
E-mail address: clea@upenn.edu

Vet Clin Small Anim 48 (2018) 751–763
https://doi.org/10.1016/j.cvsm.2018.05.009
vetsmall.theclinics.com

the development of minimally invasive therapeutic interventions and led to the creation of IR. This specialty has since grown at an exponential rate, owing to the expertise developed and advances in imaging modalities, techniques, and instrumentation.

The specialty of veterinary IR was more recently developed, applying techniques initially described in human medicine. In 2005, the first IR service was established by Dr. Chick Weisse at School of Veterinary Meicine of the University of Pennsylvania.[5] Since that time, innumerous advances have been made in this specialty, allowing the development of techniques and instrumentation, as well as an expanding number of conditions amenable to minimally invasive treatment and correction. Veterinary IR diagnostic and therapeutic procedures are performed by highly trained specialists and require proper equipment and knowledge of basic instrumentation. This article describes the equipment and techniques commonly used in veterinary IR. A more comprehensive description is available elsewhere.[6,7]

EQUIPMENT
Digital Fluoroscopy

The use of digital fluoroscopy is essential for most procedures performed in veterinary IR. Mobile C-arm digital fluoroscopy systems are used in most veterinary hospitals. Newer generations of C-arm units include the latest technology, such as flat-panel thin-film-transistor arrays, offering greater capabilities and image quality, while reducing radiation exposure. Most of these newer units are also floor- or ceiling-mounted, enabling effortless manipulations to get various projection angles. Digital fluoroscopy permits rapid acquisition of x-ray–based images as an analog video signal, which is then converted into a digital format and real-time images are projected into a monitor.[8] The images obtained can be manipulated in several ways, with digital fluoroscopy offering features such as digital subtraction angiography (DSA), road mapping, and magnification. DSA is a method in which the background of an initial non-contrast image is subtracted from subsequent serial images obtained during contrast injection to enhance the visualization of vessels after opacification with contrast (**Fig. 1**). The quality and diagnostic utility of DSA is greatly

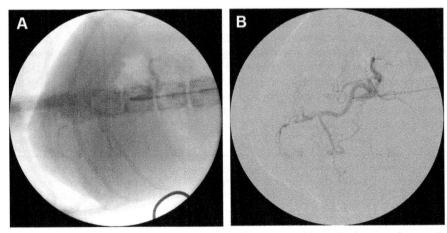

Fig. 1. Angiographic study in a dog. (*A*) Standard angiographic study showing the arterial vascularization of a liver tumor during injection of iodinated contrast medium. (*B*) Same angiographic study showing the arterial vascularization of a liver tumor during injection of iodinated contrast medium in subtraction mode. In this mode the background is subtracted and the visualization of vessels after opacification with contrast is enhanced.

affected by motion, such as respiration or heart beats, during acquisition of the images, requiring the induction of temporary apnea during most angiographic studies. Road mapping is a variation of DSA used to create a road map of the vessels of interest. Using this technique, an angiogram is performed and the image at peak opacification of the vessels is used as a mask during the acquisition of subsequent subtraction images. Using the road map created, guidewires and catheters can then be advanced and manipulated in the area studied, without the need for additional contrast injections.[5,6,8]

Some degree of exposure to radiation is unavoidable during most fluoroscopic procedures in veterinary medicine and all personnel should wear adequate protective equipment at all times. Techniques to reduce operator exposure and scatter can help limit radiation doses for those routinely performing fluoroscopic procedures. Strategies to improve radiation safety are discussed later.

Access Needles

All percutaneous endovascular procedures begin with establishment of vascular access with the use of access needles or over-the-needle catheters. A variety of vascular access needles exists, but all have a central lumen, which allows the passage of a guidewire. The size of needles is described by gauge numbers, which correspond with their outer diameter. The Seldinger needle is composed of a thin-walled outer cannula and a fitted stylet with a beveled point that is used for the double-wall puncture vascular access technique. The single-wall needle is more commonly used. It is composed of a thin-walled beveled cannula and is used for the single-wall puncture vascular access technique. Mini access kits (**Fig. 2**), also called micropuncture sets, are used to access small vessels and are therefore often beneficial when establishing vascular access in small veterinary patients. The sets include a 21-gauge needle, a 0.018″ guidewire, and a 4-Fr or 5-Fr coaxial introducer/dilator. They allow subsequent placement of larger-diameter guidewires (0.035″ or 0.038″) into the vessel after dilation from an initial small needle stick.[6,8] Users should be familiar with the access needle size and the corresponding guidewire sizes that the needle will accommodate (**Table 1**).

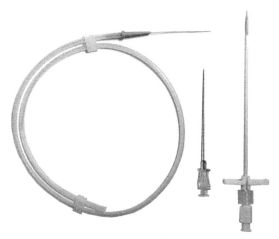

Fig. 2. Mini access kit. It includes a 21-gauge needle, a 0.018″ guidewire, and a 4-Fr or 5-Fr coaxial introducer/dilator.

Table 1 General guidelines for intravenous catheter gauge and corresponding wire sizes	
Intravenous Catheter Size	Guidewire Size
24 g	$\leq$0.018
22 g	$\leq$0.018
20 g	$\leq$0.025
18 g	$\leq$0.035
16 g	$\leq$0.038

Introducer Sheaths

Angiograms and vascular procedures are commonly performed through vascular introducer sheaths (**Fig. 3**). They are placed to maintain vascular access, protect the vessel entry site, and allow the easy and safe passage and manipulation of various guidewires and catheters through their lumens. The introducer sheath kit is composed of a beveled thin-walled outer sheath with a hemostasis valve and a side port attached at one end, and an inner thick-walled dilator that tapers to the outside diameter of the guidewire, which, depending on the brand used, may or may not contain a guidewire. Sheath and dilator sizes are described in French (Fr) and every 1 Fr corresponds to 3 mm. Sheath sizes are named for their inner diameter, as opposed to dilators and diagnostic catheters, which are named for their outer diameter. Introducer sheaths come in various lengths and sizes, and are chosen based on patient size, type of procedure performed, and the size of catheters or devices to be passed through the vascular sheath. They are placed into the vessel over a guidewire following vascular access with an access needle or an over-the-needle catheter.[6,8]

Guidewires

Guidewires are advanced and manipulated to gain access to a specific location and provide support to introduce catheters and other devices. They are radiopaque and are manipulated under fluoroscopic guidance. Various guidewires are commercially available and each have specific characteristics, such as their stiffness, coating, and tip configuration. Their size is described in hundredths of an inch, which correspond to their outer diameter. Guidewires are selected based on the inner diameter of the catheters or other devices that will be advanced over them. Guidewires of 0.035" diameter with a length of 150 cm are most commonly used in veterinary IR applications. They are made of a central stiff core around which a smaller wire is

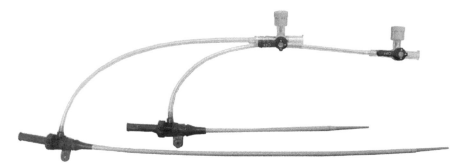

Fig. 3. Introducer sheaths.

wrapped. Most guidewires are coated with polytetrafluoroethylene (Teflon) and heparin. Some wires have a hydrophilic coating, giving them a very low coefficient of friction and making them highly resistant to kinking. The stiffness of a guidewire depends on its core thickness and composition, and the softness of the leading tip of the wire depends on the presence or absence of the central core and the length of taper of the central core at the tip. The leading tip of a guidewire is not only characterized by its softness but also by its shape, which can be angled, straight, or J shaped.[5,6,8]

Angiographic Catheters

Angiographic catheters are used to deliver radiopaque contrast media or therapeutic agents to a specific location within the body system being treated. They have a Luer adaptor at their distal end to allow the connection of syringes or other accessories. They are radiopaque and are manipulated over a guidewire to the desired location under fluoroscopic guidance. A large variety of catheters are available and their composition, coating, stiffness, inner and outer diameters, tip shape, as well as their side-hole conformation give them unique properties and are important characteristics to consider when choosing a catheter for a specific use (**Fig. 4**). They are also classified as selective or nonselective. Selective angiographic catheters are shaped to allow for catheterization of branches off the main vessel, have a thin wall for smaller-volume injections, and most have a single end hole. Nonselective angiographic catheters have a thicker wall and can handle large-volume injections, have a straight or curled tip, and have multiple side holes near the end hole to create a cloud of contrast on injection. The size of angiographic catheters is described in French (Fr), which correspond to their outer diameter, as well as in centimeters, which correspond to their length. Angiographic catheters of 4 Fr and 5 Fr are most commonly used in veterinary IR applications. The size of the vascular sheath (based on inner diameter of the sheath) through which the catheter will be advanced needs to be equal to or bigger than the size of the catheter used. For example, a 4-Fr vascular sheath will accommodate a 4-Fr angiographic catheter.[6,8]

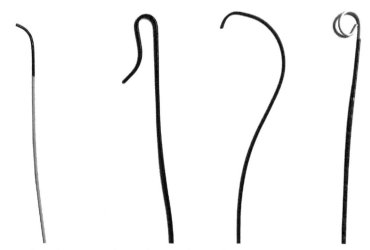

Fig. 4. Examples of angiographic catheters (from left to right: Berenstein catheter, Sidewinder catheter, Cobra 2 catheter, pigtail sizing catheter).

Balloon Dilation Catheters

Balloon dilation catheters (**Fig. 5**) are double-lumen catheters used for the dilation of stenosis or strictures of lumens (eg, urethra, nasopharynx, vessel), cardiac valves, or orifices (eg, ureterovesicular junction). They consist of 4 main parts: a double Luer lock, a shaft, the balloon, and the tip. Balloon catheters are manipulated over a guidewire under fluoroscopic guidance, and radiopaque markers are present on either end of the balloon to allow for precise positioning of the device. They are available in a range of sizes to accommodate the patient and stricture sizes. Balloon diameters are expressed in millimeters and lengths in centimeters. The size of the shaft is expressed in French, which correspond to its outer diameter, and in centimeters, which correspond to its length. Each balloon catheter has a minimum channel size, recommended guidewire size, and balloon maximum inflation pressure expressed in atmospheres. The balloon can rupture when inflated beyond its maximum inflation pressure, also termed burst pressure. Manual inflation of the balloon can be performed, but the use of an inflation device is recommended to allow for precise and controlled pressure application to the balloon. The balloon should be centered on the waist of the stricture to maximize radial force. The balloon is not radiopaque but a mixture of saline and an iodinated contrast agent is used for inflation of the balloon to visualize its position and the waist of the stricture under fluoroscopic guidance.[6,8] For vascular procedures, it is imperative that all air is cleared from the balloon before inflation in the event of accidental balloon rupture, which could result in an air embolus.

Coils and Occlusion Devices

Coils (**Fig. 6**) and occlusion devices are used in endovascular IR to reduce or obliterate blood flow through vessels, fistulae, or cardiac septal communications. Older-generation coils were made of stainless steel. Newer-generation coils are made of platinum or nickel alloy and are MRI safe. Various diameters, lengths, and shapes of coils are available. Their diameter is described in millimeters and their lengths in centimeters. Most are covered with synthetic fibers, such as Dacron, that favor thrombogenesis following deployment. Coils are radiopaque and are delivered to the desired area under fluoroscopic guidance. They are loaded into the lumen of an angiographic catheter and pushed along the shaft and out the tip of the catheter with the help of a guidewire. Occlusion devices are made of nitinol and are available in various sizes and shapes. They are used in cardiac interventions, such as persistent ductus arteriosus correction.

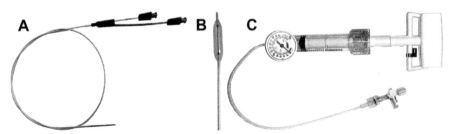

Fig. 5. Balloon dilation catheter. (*A*) Balloon dilation catheters are made of a double Luer lock, a shaft, the balloon, and the tip. (*B*) Inflated balloon. (*C*) Inflation device used for balloon inflation.

Fig. 6. Example of a coil used in angiographic procedures. Various diameters, lengths, and shapes of coils are available. They are radiopaque and are delivered to the desired area under fluoroscopic guidance.

Stents

Stents are tubular devices that are used to maintain luminal patency of vessels or other anatomic structures (eg, ureter, urethra, nasopharynx, trachea). Metallic stents are made of nitinol or stainless steel alloy and are categorized as self-expanding and balloon-expandable stents. Balloon-expandable stents are designed to allow the simultaneous dilatation of a stenosis and placement of a stent. They are mounted on a balloon catheter and expand on inflation of the balloon. They are mostly used for the treatment of nasopharyngeal stenosis,[9] but their use has also been reported for stenting of the right ventricular outflow tract,[10] treatment of Budd-Chiari–like syndrome,[11] and to relieve malignant obstructions.[12] They can be positioned precisely but can be deformed irreversibly by compressive external forces in excess of their yield point.

Self-expendable stents (**Fig. 7**) are constrained under a sheath on a low-profile delivery system and retraction of the sheath allows expansion of the stent. They are most commonly placed within the trachea, urethra, and within blood vessels.[5] They are further divided into laser-cut and woven self-expandable stents. Laser-cut stents are generally nonreconstrainable, meaning they cannot be reconstrained into the delivery system once deployment is initiated. They also have minimal foreshortening during deployment, therefore the length of the stent when implanted is the same as its manufactured length. Woven stents are most often reconstrainable, although nonreconstrainable versions also exist, so the operator must confirm reconstrainability before placement. Another property of woven stents is that they foreshorten, which causes shortening of the length of the stent as it expands. Reconstrainable stents offer flexibility during placement because they can be reconstrained into the delivery system and repositioned, as long as they have not been unsheathed beyond the limit marker band (affectionately known as the point of no return) on the delivery system.

Ureteral stents are made of radiopaque polyurethrane and have a double-coil configuration at each end and a variable numbers of side fenestrations along the length of the stent. The internal lumen is sized to accommodate standard-sized wires (0.018″-0.038″). An open-ended catheter is often provided with the stent to facilitate ureteral dilation using the tapered end of the open-ended catheter and pushing the stent into position with the nontapered end. The end coils are straightened over the wire for placement and positioning and then resume their coiled

A   **B**

Fig. 7. Self-expandable stent. (*A*) Sheath partially retracted and stent partially deployed. (*B*) Stent fully deployed following complete retraction of the sheath from the delivery system.

shape once the wire is retracted. The coils are designed to prevent stent migration, with one coil positioned within the renal pelvis and the other positioned within the bladder.

RADIATION SAFETY

As minimally invasive procedures become more widely available and routinely performed in veterinary medicine, the use of fluoroscopy will continue to grow, especially in patient care areas outside of the radiology department and by those who are not formally trained in radiology. The real-time radiographic images generated by fluoroscopy facilitate diagnostic and therapeutic interventions but carry with them the negative trade-off of ionizing radiation exposure to those performing and assisting with the procedure, the operating room staff, and the patient.[13–16]

Radiation exposure is highly regulated both on the state and federal level because of the known detrimental effects to operator and patient health. The negative consequences of radiation can be divided into 2 categories. The first is stochastic effects, which are those for which there is no defined relationship between the amount of radiation delivered and severity of the resultant injury, and include genetic mutations and neoplasia.[14] The second category is deterministic effects, which are those for which the severity of injury is associated with the received dose, and include radiation-induced skin injury and cataracts.[14] In human patients undergoing repeated procedures over the same area, those that are obese or are diabetic have increased risk of deterministic effects.[13,17–19] Radiation's biological effects, threshold doses, and time needed for recognition of negative impact on human organs have been described by the International Commission of Radiation Protection.[16–19] Fluoroscopic radiation exposure in human patients undergoing diagnostic and interventional procedures has been associated with cutaneous consequences such as hyperpigmentation, acute burns, ulceration, and delayed ulcers, as well as systemic consequences such as an increased risk of cancer.[19–23]

It is important to differentiate patient dose from exposure; patient dose is the amount of energy absorbed by the patient and exposure is the amount of radiation produced by a radiation source.[14,24] Factors that contribute to increased patient dose include backscatter, collimation, patient position, beam energy, and magnification.[14,24] In general, fluoroscopy time is considered to be the most important component of radiation exposure, although settings such as pulsed versus continuous fluoroscopy and digital subtraction also contribute to exposure.[14,24,25] At present, the best estimation of patient radiation dose is determined using 4 dose metrics that account for both dose absorbed by the skin and internal organs.[24] The 4 components of total patient dose are fluoroscopy time, peak skin dose, reference dose, and kerma-area product.[24]

Studies investigating radiation exposure in veterinary medicine, especially with regard to fluoroscopy, are lacking. Studies evaluating the risk of excess radiation doses delivered to nearby tissues during radiation planned with computed tomography (CT) and adverse radiation effects associated with radiation therapy are reported for dogs.[26–29] Results of these studies show that radiation doses during CT were below recognized thresholds.[26] However, radiation therapy for treatment of canine head and neck tumors has been documented to cause radiation injury to nontarget tissues such as the eyes, oral mucous membranes, and nearby skin.[26,28,29] Because operators must be present during fluoroscopic interventional procedures, both the patient and operator are exposed to ionizing radiation, which is in contrast with CT and radiation therapy, during which operators are not present in the room during the diagnostic or therapeutic procedure.[30,31] With the extensive knowledge of adverse radiation effects in human patients and the increase in the use of fluoroscopy in veterinary medicine, there is an imperative need for the evaluation of how fluoroscopic procedures and the associated levels of radiation exposure affect patients, clinicians, and support staff.[21,32]

A recent abstract describing 360 fluoroscopic procedures performed at 2 academic institutions where intraoperative fluoroscopy for interventional, cardiac, and orthopedic procedures are routinely performed reported C-arm data on fluoroscopy time and radiation dose.[33] Procedures were classified as vascular, urinary, respiratory, cardiac, GI, and orthopedic. Fluoroscopy operators were classified as IR trained, orthopedic surgeons, soft tissue surgeons, internists, and cardiologists. Vascular procedures had significantly longer fluoroscopy times (median 35.8 min, range 0.6–84.7 min) and significantly higher radiation dose (median 137 mGy, range 13–617.5 mGy) than urinary, GI, orthopedic, cardiac, and respiratory procedures ($P = .001$). Trained interventional radiologists (16.1 mGy) and cardiologists (25.8 mGy) were associated with significantly higher radiation exposure than any other operators ($P = .001$).[33] This study demonstrated that vascular procedures were associated with significantly longer fluoroscopic times and higher radiation exposure than other fluoroscopic procedures evaluated. In the human literature, vascular procedures, such as transjugular intrahepatic portosystemic shunt (TIPS) creation and embolization of aneurysms and arteriovenous malformations, are also associated with higher radiation exposure and are typically classified as high-dose procedures.[34] Many human vascular interventional procedures routinely exceed a patient radiation dose of 2 Gy, which is the threshold determined by the International Commission on Radiological Protection for deterministic effects.[35]

There are several reasons why vascular interventional procedures are associated with higher radiation exposure, including the high level of detail needed to visualize small or complex vasculature, use of DSA and road mapping, magnification, and increased total fluoroscopy time. Settings to reduce exposure, such as lower frame rate, pulsed fluoroscopy, low fluoroscopy dose settings, and collimation, reduce radiation received by the patient but may compromise visualization and image quality.[25,36] During endovascular aneurysm repair using a mobile C arm, low-dose and pulsed fluoroscopy modes significantly reduced patient radiation dose compared with standard C-arm settings.[25] Newer C-arm technology to optimize acquisition parameters and real-time processing has also been shown to significantly reduce patient radiation exposure during intra-arterial chemoembolization of nonresectable liver tumors in people.[35] Educational training programs for fluoroscopic operators have documented improved understanding of fluoroscopic safety principles, produce higher quality imaging, and reduce total fluoroscopy time and radiation exposure.[36–38]

Ionizing radiation exposure to both patients and operators is associated with 3 main factors: time, distance, and intensity. Even though there are no reports of fluoroscopy-induced radiation injury in small animals, techniques to minimize procedure time, use of lowest possible fluoroscopic dose possible while still achieving adequate image quality to complete the procedure safely, collimation, magnification, and x-ray beam geometry can help limit patient and operator exposure. High-dose settings, such as HQ (high quality) and DSA, and high frame rates should only be used when necessary, such as for angiographic studies or device deployment, and not for catheter positioning and manipulation.[14] Many fluoroscopic units are equipped with laser crosshairs that can be used to confirm appropriate tube positioning without the need for fluoroscopic guided positioning. High dose and frame rates should be avoided for low-motion areas of the body, such as extremities.[14] When considering patient distance, space between the patient and image intensifier, as well as beam geometry need to be taken into account. Patients should be positioned as far away from the x-ray tube, and as close to the image intensifier, as possible.[14] However, for procedures in small patients when the area being treated requires operator access alternating with fluoroscopic evaluation, positioning the patient close to the image intensifier can be challenging for access and dexterity. When the x-ray tube and image intensifier are vertically aligned over the patient, patient dose is reduced.[14] When the intensifier is in an oblique position over the patient, there is an increased air gap, requiring more radiation to penetrate the patient and increasing dose.[14]

When considering the fluoroscopic operator, scatter is the most significant source of exposure, therefore techniques to limit scatter are important for fluoroscopists, especially for those making a career performing interventional procedures during which they are routinely exposed over years. Angulation of the tube toward the operator increases their radiation exposure.[14] Because radiation exposure is defined by the inverse square law, doubling the distance from the tube decreases exposure by a factor of 4. Therefore, stepping away from the x-ray tube during the procedure as much as possible, especially during runs of continuous fluoroscopy, or being far away from the x-ray tube if not directly involved in the procedure, are simple strategies to greatly reduce radiation exposure.[14] Most scatter occurs from the patient and table, therefore lead-equivalent shields mounted on the ceiling or from articulating arm booms, or those that are on wheels, can be helpful at limiting exposure by providing versatile shielding that can be moved and positioned as indicated by the patient, procedure, or access point. Table-mounted lead-equivalent skirts can cover the x-ray tube when it is positioned under the table, thereby limiting operator exposure when they stand in close proximity of the x-ray tube. Sterile flexible bismuth drapes that can be placed over the patient have been shown to limit scatter to the operator's eye, thyroid, and hand but must not be placed in the primary beam because they cause increased radiation output if detected by the fluoroscopy unit's automatic brightness control and increase skin dose.[14,39]

Personal shielding is required of all present in the IR suite while fluoroscopy is in use. Lead-equivalent aprons, particularly those that wrap around the operator to provide complete coverage, are often the most comfortable and safe, especially if the person's back is turned during live fluoroscopy. Body gowns cover and protect the most radiosensitive organs, including lungs, GI tract, gonads, and most bone marrow.[14] Detached thyroid shields should also be worn to protect the thyroid. Years of exposure to fluoroscopic radiation can induce cataract formation, which is why protective eyewear is also recommended. It is especially important to note that the cataracts that result from prolonged radiation exposure cannot be addressed surgically; therefore, prevention is essential. All shielding should be as comfortable for the operator as possible and fit well because protective equipment that is cumbersome and uncomfortable will not be worn.[14] Care must be taken to hang the gowns properly to prevent cracking of the composite within the gowns. Ideally, to limit creasing, individuals should not sit in their gowns, which can lead to cracks and decreased shielding ability. In the past, routine fluoroscopic evaluation of gowns was recommended to evaluate for cracks and gaps in the gowns so that they could be removed from use. However, more recent recommendations are to carefully palpate the gowns for cracks and creases, and take a radiograph of the area of concern to limit additional fluoroscopic exposure.

Sterile radiation-attenuating gloves can be used but decrease dexterity and may not significantly reduce hand exposure from scatter and do not provide protection against direct beam exposure.[14,40] Dosimetry requirements vary by state, but most require placement of dosimeter badges on an outer gown pocket or at the level of the thyroid. Ring badges provide information regarding radiation exposure to the hands and should also be worn for all fluoroscopic procedures. They can be soaked in glutaraldehyde cold sterile solutions such as Cidex so that they can be worn under sterile gloves for procedures requiring asepsis.

REFERENCES

1. Murphy TP, Soares GM. The evolution of interventional radiology. Semin Intervent Radiol 2005;22:6–9.
2. Murphy TP. Introduction to clinical interventional radiology. Semin Intervent Radiol 2005;22:3–5.
3. Seldinger SI. Catheter replacement of the needle in percutaneous arteriography; a new technique. Acta Radiol 1953;39:368–76.
4. Dotter CT, Judkins MP. Transluminal treatment of arteriosclerotic obstruction. Description of a new technic and a preliminary report of its application. Circulation 1964;30:654–70.
5. Scansen BA. Interventional radiology equipment and techniques. Vet Clin North Am Small Anim Pract 2016;46:535–52.
6. Sun F. Tools of the trade – interventional radiology. In: Weisse C, Berent A, editors. Veterinary image-guided interventions. Ames (IA): Wiley-Blackwell; 2015. p. 3–14.
7. Berent AC. Tools of the trade – interventional endoscopy. In: Weisse C, Berent A, editors. Veterinary image-guided interventions. Ames (IA): Wiley-Blackwell; 2015. p. 15–28.
8. Kaufman JA. Fundamentals of angiography. In: Kaufman JA, Lee MJ, editors. Vascular and interventional radiology: the requisites. 2nd edition. Philadelphia: Elsevier Saunders; 2014. p. 25–55.
9. Bird L, Nelissen P, White RA, et al. Treatment of canine nasopharyngeal stenosis using balloon-expandable metallic stents: long-term follow-up of four cases. J Small Anim Pract 2016;57:265–70.
10. Scansen BA, Kent AM, Cheatham SL, et al. Stenting of the right ventricular outflow tract in 2 dogs for palliation of dysplastic pulmonary valve stenosis and right-to-left intracardiac shunting defects. J Vet Cardiol 2014;16:205–14.
11. Hoehne SN, Milovancev M, Hyde AJ, et al. Placement of a caudal vena cava stent for treatment of Budd-Chiari-like syndrome in a 4-month-old Ragdoll cat. J Am Vet Med Assoc 2014;245:414–8.
12. Newman RG, Mehler SJ, Kitchell BE, et al. Use of a balloon-expandable metallic stent to relieve malignant urethral obstruction in a cat. J Am Vet Med Assoc 2009; 234:236–9.
13. Weisse CW, Berent AC, Todd KL, et al. Potential applications of interventional radiology in veterinary medicine. J Am Vet Med Assoc 2008;233(10):1564–7.
14. Marx MV. Radiation safety and protection in the interventional fluoroscopy environment. In: Mauro MA, Murphy KP, Thompson KR, et al, editors. Image-guided interventions (a volume in the expert radiology series). Philadelphia: Elsevier; 2014. p. 59–62.
15. Weisse C. Veterinary interventional oncology: from concept to clinic. Vet J 2015; 205(2):198–203.
16. Weisse C. Introduction to interventional radiology for the criticalist. J Vet Emerg Crit Care (San Antonio) 2011;21(2):79–85.

17. Stewart FA, Akleyev AV, Hauer-Jensen M, et al. ICRP PUBLICATION 118: ICRP Statement on tissue reactions and early and late effects of radiation in normal tissues and organs – threshold doses for tissue reactions in a radiation protection context. Ann ICRP 2012;41(1–2):1–322.

18. Goodhead DT. Understanding and characterization of the risks to human health from exposure to low levels of radiation. Radiat Prot Dosimetry 2009;137(1): 109–17.

19. Wagner LK, McNeese MD, Marx MV, et al. Severe skin reactions from interventional fluoroscopy: case report and review of the literature. Radiology 1999; 213(3):773–6.

20. Koenig TR, Mettler FA, Wagner LK. Skin injuries from fluoroscopically guided procedures: part 2, review of 73 cases and recommendations for minimizing dose delivered to patient. AJR Am J Roentgenol 2001;177:13–20.

21. Valentin J. Avoidance of radiation injuries from medical interventional procedures. ICRP publication 85. Ann ICRP 2000;30(2):7–67.

22. Boice JD Jr, Preston D, Davis FG, et al. Frequent chest X-ray fluoroscopy and breast cancer incidence among tuberculosis patients in Massachusetts. Radiat Res 1991;125(2):214–22.

23. Hunter N, Muirhead CR, González AJ, et al. radiation Uncertainties in estimating health risks associated with exposure to ionising radiation. J Radiol Prot 2013;33: 573–88.

24. Jaco JW, Miller DL. Measuring and monitoring radiation dose during fluoroscopically guided procedures. Tech Vasc Interv Radiol 2010;13(3):188–93.

25. Maurel B, Sobocinski J, Perini P, et al. Evaluation of radiation during EVAR performed on a mobile C-arm. Eur J Vasc Endovasc Surg 2012;43(1):16–21.

26. Yoshikawa H, Roback DM, Larue SM, et al. Stereotactic body radiotherapy planning. Vet Radiol Ultrasound 2015;56(6):687–95.

27. Xu W, Chen J, Xu L, et al. Acute radiation enteritis caused by dose-dependent radiation exposure in dogs: experimental research. Exp Biol Med (Maywood) 2014;239:1543–56.

28. Hunley DW, Mauldin GN, Shiomitsu K, et al. Clinical outcome in dogs with nasal tumors treated with intensity-modulated radiation therapy. Can Vet J 2010;51: 293–300.

29. Ching SV, Gillette SM, Powers BE, et al. Radiation-induced ocular injury in the dog: a histological study. Int J Radiat Oncol Biol Phys 1990;19:321–8.

30. Goodman BS, Carnel CT, Mallempati S, et al. Reduction in average fluoroscopic exposure times for interventional spinal procedures through the use of pulsed and low-dose image settings. Am J Phys Med Rehabil 2011;90(11):908–12.

31. Shortt CP, Al-Hashimi H, Malone L, et al. Staff radiation doses to the lower extremities in interventional radiology. Cardiovasc Intervent Radiol 2007;30(6):1206–9.

32. Hersh-Boyle R, Culp W, Brown D, et al. Evaluation of patient radiation exposure in veterinary procedure utilizing intra-operative fluoroscopy: 360 cases. Proceedings of the Veterinary Interventional Radiology & Interventional Endoscopy Society (VIRIES), Jackson Hole, WY, June 13-15, 2016.

33. Miller DL, Balter S, Cole PE, et al. Radiation doses in interventional radiology procedures: the RAD-IR study part I: overall measures of dose radiation doses in interventional radiology procedures: part I. J Vasc Interv Radiol 2003;14:711–27.

34. Cho JH, Kim JY, Kang JE, et al. A study to compare the radiation absorbed dose of the C-arm fluoroscopic modes. Korean J Pain 2011;24(4):199–204.

35. Schernthaner RE, Duran R, Chapiro J, et al. A new angiographic imaging platform reduces radiation exposure for patients with liver cancer treated with

transarterial chemoembolization. Eur Radiol 2015;3255–62. https://doi.org/10.1007/s00330-015-3717-0.

36. Kirkwood ML, Arbique GM, Guild JB, et al. Surgeon education decreases radiation dose in complex endovascular procedures and improves patient safety. J Vasc Surg 2013;58(3):715–21.

37. Bar-On E, Weigl DM, Becker T, et al. Intraoperative C-arm radiation affecting factors and reduction by an intervention program. J Pediatr Orthop 2010;30(4):320–3.

38. Bott OJ, Dresing K, Wagner M, et al. Informatics in radiology: use of a C-arm fluoroscopy simulator to support training in intraoperative radiography. Radiographics 2011;31:E64–74.

39. King JN, Champlin AM, Kelsey CA, et al. Using a sterile disposable protective surgical drape for reduction of radiation exposure to interventionalists. AJR Am J Roentgenol 2002;178:153–7.

40. Wagner LK, Mulhern OR. Radiation-attenuating surgical gloves: effects of scatter and secondary electron production. Radiology 1996;200:45–8.

Interventional Radiology Management of Tracheal and Bronchial Collapse

Dana L. Clarke, VMD

KEYWORDS

- Tracheal collapse • Chondromalacia • Honking • Extraluminal prosthetic rings
- Tracheal stent • Fluoroscopy

KEY POINTS

- Tracheal and bronchial collapse are common causes of coughing and upper airway obstructions in small-breed dogs.
- Fluoroscopy provides dynamic noninvasive assessment of airway diameter changes during normal respiration and coughing to help confirm the diagnosis without general anesthesia.
- When medical management fails to control a patient's clinical signs and alleviate upper airway obstruction, tracheal stenting provides a minimally invasive rapid treatment to restore airway patency.
- Tracheal stent placement under fluoroscopy provides real-time dynamic feedback about stent positioning in the airway and degree of opening so that it can be reconstrained and repositioned if needed.

INTRODUCTION

Tracheal collapse is a common, frustrating disease process in small-breed dogs that results from progressive degeneration of the airway cartilages secondary to chondromalacia.[1–6] Collapse of the airway cartilages and repeated luminal contact results in chronic inflammation, which precipitates further coughing, leading to worsened inflammation, and perpetuation of a vicious cycle of cough and inflammation. The persistent tracheal inflammation also causes loss of the columnated ciliary epithelial component of the mucociliary escalator, leading to squamous metaplasia. Loss of ciliary function also causes coughing to become the major mechanism of tracheobronchial clearance, adding to the vicious cycle of coughing and inflammation.[1–4,6] Bronchomalacia is a similar change to the cartilages of the bronchi and bronchioles. It can occur as an isolated syndrome or in conjunction with tracheal collapse and can affect dogs of all sizes.[7–10]

Department of Clinical Sciences and Advanced Medicine, University of Pennsylvania School of Veterinary Medicine, Philadelphia, PA 19104, USA
E-mail address: clarked@vet.upenn.edu

Vet Clin Small Anim 48 (2018) 765–779
https://doi.org/10.1016/j.cvsm.2018.05.010
0195-5616/18/© 2018 Elsevier Inc. All rights reserved.

Signalment, history, and physical examination findings can support a tentative diagnosis of tracheobronchial collapse, but localization of the disease along the trachea and lower airways requires targeted client questions and diagnostic imaging. Once the extent and severity of disease are understood, medical management should be implemented in all cases except those so severely affected that discharge without intervention is not possible. Tracheal stenting has become a popular, noninvasive method for treating tracheal collapse in dogs. Initial experience with tracheal stenting was met with significant complications, leading to it being branded a salvage procedure. Design enhancements, progress in sizing protocols, and improved patient selection criteria have increased the success of their use.

HISTORY, CLINICAL SIGNS, AND PHYSICAL EXAMINATION FINDINGS

A thorough history and physical examination are essential in all dogs presented for tracheal collapse evaluation, because many dogs have compromise of multiple locations in the upper airway, including the nasopharynx, larynx, trachea, and bronchi. In addition to a complete medical history, pointed questions directed to disease localization and severity are important to determine airway obstruction from lower airway and pulmonary parenchymal disease (**Box 1**).

Visual assessment of the patient breathing at rest, during respiratory noise and/or coughing, is needed to evaluate for the nature of the cough, prolongation of inspiratory or expiratory phase of respiration, increased respiratory effort, abdominal push on expiration, and herniation of the cranial lung lobes out of the thoracic inlet on expiration or during coughing episodes. Auditory assessment from a distance should assess for the nature of abnormal respiratory noises (honking, high pitched, wheezing moist, stertor, or stridor). The larynx, trachea, and entire thorax should be carefully auscultated with simultaneous observation of respiratory phase for air movement, fluid sounds in the large airways, wheezes, and crackles. The presence of an inducible cough on tracheal palpation is not pathognomonic for tracheal collapse because aggressive palpation can induce patients with normal tracheas to cough.

Box 1
Questions to help differentiate airway obstruction from lower airway and pulmonary parenchymal disease

1. Duration and progression of clinical signs

2. Past treatments administered and response to therapy

3. Nature of respiratory noise (honking, dry hacking cough, soft cough, moist/productive cough, expiratory wheezing, terminal retch, gagging)

4. How frequent are events and how long do they last

5. Does the pet appear to have respiratory difficulty or distress during or after an event

6. What are the triggers for a coughing or respiratory event

7. Is the pet able to sleep through the night without coughing

8. Does the pet snore or have signs of airway obstruction when sleeping

9. Is there a seasonal component to the respiratory events

10. What is the home environment like (is there smoking, air conditioning, air fresheners, and the like)

Tracheal collapse, which is isolated to the cervical trachea, causes increased inspiratory respiratory effort and noise due to the weakened airway's inability to withstand negative intraluminal pressure generated on inspiration. Tracheal collapse isolated to the intrathoracic portion of the trachea results in expiratory noise and effort due to airway collapse from an inability to withstand increased thoracic pressures upon exhalation. Collapse at the thoracic inlet may cause either or both inspiratory and expiratory signs. Bronchial collapse is common in dogs with tracheal collapse and has been documented in 83% of dogs with cervical tracheal collapse.[7,11] The location of airway narrowing, as well as the presence or absence of concurrent bronchial collapse, determines the clinical signs and severity of respiratory compromise.

The author finds most dogs presented for tracheal collapse evaluation can be classified as "honkers" and "coughers," although there are some dogs that have characteristics of both classes. The classic "honking" noise heard with respiration and panting is typically seen with obstructive airway disease, generally with collapse of the cervical or thoracic inlet trachea. The severity of the honk can be exacerbated by stress, activity, and excitement. Other signs of airway obstruction include stridor, stertor, gagging after eating and drinking, and exercise intolerance.[1,3,11,12] Conversely, pure coughing dogs tend to have a dry, hacking cough, which can also be high pitched and may or may not be productive.[7–9] These dogs do not tend to have exercise intolerance or respiratory distress when mildly to moderately affected, but can with more advanced disease or concurrent pulmonary parenchymal disease. Coughing tends to be the result of bronchial collapse, pulmonary parenchymal disease, and/or intrathoracic tracheal collapse. Many patients will have components of both coughing and obstruction, and determination of the primary problem can help guide diagnostics and therapy.

Additional physical examination findings common in dogs with airway obstruction (honking) versus those with lower airway disease (coughing) as their primary problem are outlined in **Table 1**.

DIAGNOSTIC TESTING

Because many patients with tracheobronchial collapse can have impaired respiratory function, concurrent pneumonia, or other pulmonary parenchymal disease, assessment of adequate oxygenation and ventilation is important, especially in patients presenting

Table 1
Physical examination findings that may be noted in dogs with airway obstruction as their primary source of respiratory compromise (honkers) and those with lower airway disease, such as bronchial collapse, chronic bronchitis, and/or intrathoracic tracheal collapse (coughers) primarily affecting their airway

"Honkers"	"Coughers"
Abducted elbows	Increased respiratory effort on expiration
Prolonged inspiratory phase of respiration	Expiratory abdominal "push"
Increased respiratory effort on inspiration	Harsh expiratory lung sounds
Pectus excavatum	Herniation of cranial lung lobes
Sinus arrhythmia	Crackles on pulmonary auscultation
External rotation of the costochrondral junctions creating pointed ventral ribs	Overdeveloped abdominal musculature creating a "heave line"
Extended head/neck/orthopnea	Perineal hernia
Increased or decreased sounds on cervical/thoracic inlet tracheal auscultation	Fecal incontinence from increased abdominal pressure on coughing expiration

in respiratory distress. Pulse oximetry, venous blood-gas analysis for ventilation assessment, or arterial blood-gas analysis for determination of both oxygenation and ventilation should be considered in all patients presenting for respiratory evaluation.

Three-view thoracic radiographs, ideally including the cervical neck and larynx, should be performed in all patients with suspected tracheobronchial collapse. Because tracheal collapse is a dynamic disease process, it can be missed or underestimated on radiographs, even with paired inspiratory and expiratory radiographs.[13] When compared with fluoroscopy, a study evaluating the utility of paired inspiratory and expiratory radiographs showed that the location of collapse was misdiagnosed in 44% of dogs and even failed to diagnose tracheal collapse in 8% of dogs.[13] Thoracic radiographs may also underestimate the presence or degree of bronchial collapse as well as create the appearance of worsened bronchointerstitial lung disease if only expiratory films are obtained. Irrespective of their shortcomings for dynamic airway diameter changes, they are essential to evaluate for bronchopneumonia, bronchial and/or interstitial lung disease, the size of cardiovascular structures, mediastinal changes, and pulmonary neoplasia. To more thoroughly assess for dynamic tracheal and bronchial diameter changes during all phases of respiration, lung lobe herniation, and dynamic nasopharyngeal collapse, awake fluoroscopy is preferred to globally assess the airway and avoid the need for general anesthesia (**Fig. 1**).[14,15] Computed tomography (CT) can also be used for dynamic airway assessment in awake or lightly sedated patients when a plastic patient positioning device (MouseTrap) is used to restrict patient movement and provide supplemental oxygen if needed (**Fig. 2**).[16] If CT is used to determine tracheal stent sizing, intubation and positive pressure ventilation are needed as for radiographic or fluoroscopic stent sizing (see later discussion).[17]

In dogs with coughing as their primary complaint, especially if there is concern for chronic bronchitis, bronchial collapse, and/or noninfectious pulmonary parenchymal disease, echocardiography should also be considered to assess for secondary pulmonary hypertension. Patients for whom a portion of their coughing is attributable to pulmonary hypertension secondary to chronic lower airway disease may have improvement in their cough with treatment of the pulmonary hypertension.

Tracheobronchoscopy is the gold standard for evaluating and grading airway collapse, although endoscopic grade of collapse does not always correspond with severity of clinical signs.[9,11,18,19] Given concerns for recovery from general anesthesia after airway evaluation in dogs with tracheobronchial collapse, the author prefers to reserve this diagnostic for patients undergoing definitive airway intervention or those from whom the benefits of airway evaluation and sampling outweighs the risks of a

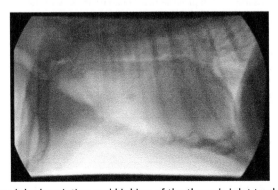

Fig. 1. Cranial lung lobe herniation and kinking of the thoracic inlet trachea during coughing in a dog with severe bronchial collapse and intrathoracic tracheal collapse.

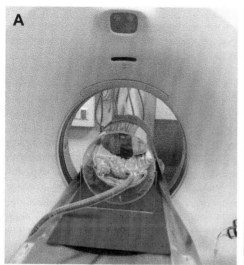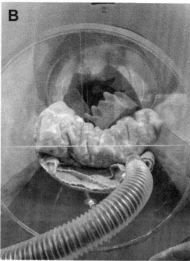

Fig. 2. VetMouseTrap. (*A*) Yorkshire Terrier restrained in the VetMouseTrap (TM) device to facilitate computed tomography (CT) of the thorax without anesthesia while being provided supplemental oxygen. (*B*) Padding placed within the device to help keep the patient in sternal recumbancy and prevent movement (Universal Medical Systems, Solon, OH).

potentially complicated anesthetic recovery. Before anesthesia for endoscopic examination, a thorough laryngeal examination for structure and function should be performed to rule out laryngeal paralysis and varying degrees of laryngeal collapse.[11,20] Airway sampling via endotracheal wash or bronchoalveolar lavage should also be considered in all dogs with suspected tracheobronchial disease undergoing general anesthesia. The trachea is not sterile, and bacterial species such as *Pasteurella*, *Staphylococcus* sp, *Streptococcus*, and *Klebsiella* have been cultured from the airway of normal dogs.[21] Therefore, cytology is important to document evidence of infection and/or inflammation with concurrent positive culture results. In dogs with tracheobronchial collapse diagnosed via endoscopy, as well as those undergoing tracheal stent placement, bacterial isolates cultured include *Pseudomonas*, *Pasteurella*, *Escherichia coli*, *Staphylococci*, and *Enterobacter aerogenes*.[19,22,23] Mycoplasma culture and polymerase chain reaction (PCR) should also be considered, although the exact role of this pathogen in tracheobronchial collapse is not fully understood.

MEDICAL MANAGEMENT

Medical therapy is the core of tracheobronchial collapse management. However, it is very important to remember that medications only control clinical signs of coughing and inflammation; they do not directly address airway collapse or obstruction. Regardless, efforts should be made to institute medical therapies before surgical or interventional options are pursued, because up to 71% of dogs can be effectively managed with medications for more than 12 months.[1] Oftentimes, "breaking the cycle" of dyspnea, distress, and anxiety with sedation, oxygen, cough suppression, and possibly corticosteroids is effective at controlling airway collapse symptoms well enough to permit discharge with medical management initiation or adjustment or referral for further intervention. The role of bronchodilators in tracheal collapse alone is controversial, although they may be indicated in patients with bronchial collapse and/or chronic bronchitis. There are cases wherein respiratory distress cannot be controlled, or there is significant patient compromise and immediate relief of the airway obstruction is needed.[24,25] For a complete discussion of medical management options and dosing, readers are directed to other references.[3,4,12]

TRACHEAL STENTING

Tracheal stenting directly addresses the physiology of collapse by supporting the dorsal tracheal membrane and weakened cartilages with 360° of intraluminal radial outward force, opening the airway from the inside. They can be placed quickly and minimally invasively, using a variety of guidance techniques, including fluoroscopy, digital radiography, or bronchoscopy. Fluoroscopy is preferred by the author because it allows for constant assessment of stent positioning, degree of opening, and evaluation of stent proximity to the absolute boundaries for placement: the cricoid cartilage cranially and the carina caudally. Measurements to determine stent size are made under general anesthesia because of relaxation of the dorsal tracheal membrane and positive pressure ventilation to maximally expand the airway. Currently, there is no method to predict the appropriate stent size before the measurements made under general anesthesia. Therefore, in critical patients who cannot recover from general anesthesia without relief of the airway obstruction, a variety of stent sizes (both length and diameter) need to be readily available for placement immediately after measurements determine the ideal size. Since most tracheal stent complications result from issues with sizing, it is imperative to size the stent as precisely as possible based on the measurements obtained. It is also extremely important to understand what can and cannot be accomplished with tracheal stenting. For dogs with airway obstruction and respiratory distress secondary to tracheal collapse, tracheal stenting is a life-saving procedure to alleviate the obstruction and improve respiratory comfort. For dogs whose only clinical sign is coughing secondary to lower airway disease and/or bronchial collapse, or those from whom most of their clinical signs are associated with coughing and not obstruction, tracheal stenting is likely to provide limited relief. Most dogs for whom tracheal stents are placed will continue to require lifelong cough suppression; therefore, emphasizing this long-term management consideration *before* stent placement helps to manage client expectations.

Candidates for tracheal stent placement are dogs that are poor candidates for surgery, such as those with existing laryngeal dysfunction, those with impaired healing concerns, or those from whom prolonged anesthesia could be detrimental, dogs whose owners are unaccepting of the risks of extraluminal ring placement, such as laryngeal paralysis, or those with intrathoracic or diffuse tracheal collapse.[1,5,22,24–31] Tracheal stents have also been shown to be beneficial in dogs with tracheal collapse that present in respiratory crisis that is nonresponsive to medical stabilization and animals with airway obstruction secondary to nonresectable tracheal masses or strictures.[24,25,32]

Initial research into tracheal stent placement in dogs was performed with balloon expandable and laser cut biliary wall stents in research dogs and clinical tracheal collapse patients. Significant complications were met with the stents and patient population chosen, including foreshortening, migration, fracture, and excessive airway inflammation.[5,20,27–29,33–36] Based on these complications, tracheal stenting was branded a salvage procedure that was to be considered only when all other medical and surgical options had been exhausted. Based on the experiences learned from complications, production of self-expanding, woven, nitinol reconstrainable stents designed specifically for canine tracheal collapse were created and have undergone multiple design enhancements to improve ease of placement and reduce risk of fracture formation (VetStent Trachea; Infiniti Medical, Menlo Park, CA, USA).

Tracheal stent measurements are made under general anesthesia, with stent placement immediately upon determination of ideal size under the same anesthetic event whenever possible. Radiographs, fluoroscopy, and CT have been described to measure anesthetized maximal tracheal diameters.[17,37] The author performs a thorough laryngeal examination for structure and function, followed by endotracheal wash and tracheoscopy in all patients before stent placement. To perform measurements for tracheal stent sizing, the patient is placed in right lateral recumbency position. A marker catheter is placed within a red rubber catheter and then advanced into the esophagus under fluoroscopic guidance. The absolute tracheal boundaries, the cricoid cartilage and the carina, are identified under fluoroscopy. In cases where the cricoid cartilage is not well mineralized, this boundary can be difficult to visualize. When this occurs, the author prefers to palpate the cricoid cartilage and place a small needle (22- to 25-g) in the lateral neck subcutaneous tissue at the level of the cartilage to create a better defined demarcation of this essential boundary (**Fig. 3**). To make measurements of the maximal tracheal diameter, a positive pressure breath is held at 20 to 30 cm H_2O using the inflated endotracheal tube cuff to maintain airway pressure. The endotracheal tube can be either positioned within the larynx, and then measurements made at several (3–6) locations along the trachea, or the endotracheal tube can be sequentially retracted from the intrathoracic trachea to the larynx, and 2 to 4 measurements made at each segment of the trachea (2–4 intrathoracic measurements, 2–4 thoracic inlet measurements, and 2–4 cervical tracheal measurements).[37,38] The author prefers the latter technique because it allows for the endotracheal tube to serve as a support for the dorsal tracheal membrane, limiting the distance needed to expand the dorsal tracheal membrane to its maximal diameter during positive pressure breath-holds.

Stent size is chosen by selecting a stent with a diameter that is 10% to 20% larger than the maximal tracheal diameter measurement obtained. Once the desired diameter is selected, length is chosen by selecting a stent that will at least cover all of the collapse and provide an additional 1 cm of stent contact cranial and caudal to the collapse. Traditionally, stent lengths were chosen to span the area of collapse only. However, given the progressive nature of tracheal collapse, most people prefer

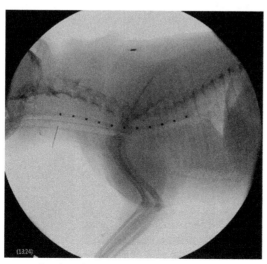

Fig. 3. Subcutaneous needle placed at the level of the cricoid cartilage to define the caudal border of the larynx during tracheal stent placement.

to span as much of the tracheal length as possible with the stent, bearing in mind the cricoid and carina absolute boundaries.

In some cases, the tracheal diameter is not uniform along its length, with the most common scenario being a larger cervical and cranial thoracic inlet diameter compared with the intrathoracic tracheal diameter (**Fig. 4**). Stent choice in these cases mandates that either the cervical trachea is undersized to accommodate the intrathoracic trachea or the thoracic trachea is oversized to accommodate the cervical trachea when using traditional tubular stents. Because accurate sizing is thought to be paramount in the success of tracheal stenting, a self-expanding, woven nitinol stent with a tapering diameter where the cervical tracheal diameter stent portion is larger than the intrathoracic portion was designed. Initial clinical case experience with the tapered tracheal stent (VetStent Duality; Infiniti Medical, Menlo Park, CA) has been very promising (see **Fig. 4**).[39] Complications seen with tracheal stenting are thought to be greatly reduced when precise sizing is performed. Oversized stents that do not fully expand are at increased risk of fracture because stents are strongest when fully expanded. Alternatively, undersized stents are at risk of migration and poor incorporation into the tracheal mucosa, leading to mucous accumulation, inflammation, and likely infection. Unequal tracheal mucosal contact, in conjunction with airway inflammation and infection, may also lead to granulomatous/inflammatory tissue formation, but objective data correlating these circumstances are lacking.

Tracheal stents are placed through an endotracheal tube with a bronchoscope adapter attached to the anesthetic circuit, which allows the patient to continue to have oxygen insufflation during stent positioning and deployment. Because the circuit will leak during stent placement, avoidance of inhaled anesthetics is advisable, and total intravenous anesthetic protocols should be considered. Constant fluoroscopic visualization during deployment ensures the caudal end of the stent remains in the desired location, the stent is expanding as expected, and that the cranial aspect of the stent is not deployed into the larynx. Care must also be taken to retract the endotracheal tube during stent deployment to ensure the opened stent is not inadvertently opened into the endotracheal tube. Most tracheal stents are reconstrainable and can be recaptured into the delivery sheath until approximately 75% of the stent is deployed. After the stent is placed in the desired position, the delivery system is carefully removed under fluoroscopy to prevent the nose-cone (tip) from inadvertently becoming caught in the stent and causing displacement.

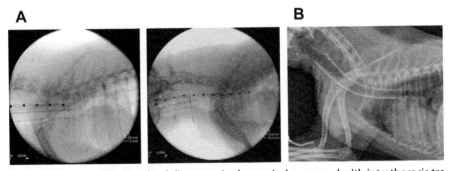

Fig. 4. Different maximal tracheal diameters in the cervical compared with intrathoracic trachea (*A*) and placement of a tapered tracheal stent (Duality) (*B*) to optimize sizing of the tracheal stent throughout its length.

Tracheoscopy is repeated after stent placement to evaluate for areas of poor contact that could become areas of incomplete mucosal ingrowth and allow mucous accumulation, chronic infections, and granulomatous tissue formation (**Fig. 5**). Should this be documented, balloon dilation of the stent can be attempted to further expand the stent and engage the mucosa. If this is still ineffective, removal of the tracheal stent and placement of a larger size or second stent may be considered. Areas of gapping/poor contact should be aggressively addressed early when the stent can be removed. Otherwise, the stent will begin to become incorporated into the mucosa within several days, after which point the stent cannot be removed. Because areas of poor contact/gapping, mucous accumulation, and chronic infection often do not become apparent for several months, the time delay to diagnosis precludes stent removal. For this reason, repeat tracheoscopy immediately after stent placement has become an invaluable aspect of successful case management.

Patients are often discharged the day after stent placement, unless there is concurrent pneumonia requiring prolonged hospital care. All tracheal stent patients have thoracic radiographs taken before discharge to confirm positioning and evaluate for pneumonia that may have developed secondary to anesthesia. Patients are discharged with antibiotics pending airway culture, a 2-to 3-week tapering course of steroids, and regular (every 6–8 hour) cough suppression. A short, dry, self-limiting cough is to be expected for 4 to 6 weeks after stent placement and represents another important aspect of postoperative stent patient care that should be discussed with the client before the procedure is performed. This conversation is especially important in dogs whose only clinical signs are airway obstruction and honking, because they will develop at least temporary coughing after stent placement, turning a noncoughing, honking dog into a nonhonking but coughing dog.

Long-term routine thoracic radiograph monitoring is important to be able to detect migration, early fracture, or the development of inflammatory tissue. For the first year after stent placement, radiographs are checked every 3 to 4 months. For every year after that, radiographs are taken every 6 months. If at any point postoperatively there is a change in the patient's cough or respiratory comfort, repeat radiographs are taken immediately. If radiographs and/or tracheal fluoroscopy do not reveal the explanation

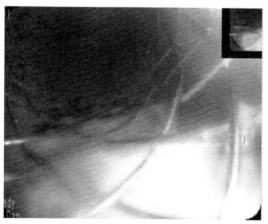

Fig. 5. Repeat tracheoscopy performed immediately after tracheal stent placement, demonstrating a gap between the tracheal stent and mucosa, which could become a source of mucous trapping and chronic infection.

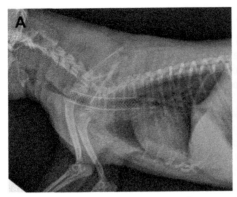
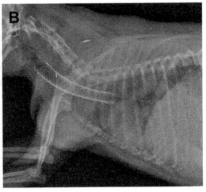

Fig. 6. Progressive cervical tracheal collapse cranial to the original stent (*A*) and placement of a second tracheal stent to address the area of progressive collapse (*B*).

for changes in coughing and respiratory comfort, repeat endotracheal wash and tracheoscopy is indicated.

TRACHEAL STENT COMPLICATIONS

Because tracheal stents are permanent implants, careful patient selection and consultation are imperative. Reported complications include stent fracture, migration, chronic infections, granulomatous/inflammatory tissue, and progressive collapse in unstented regions of the trachea. With appropriate sizing, stent migration is very uncommon and generally occurs soon after stent implantation before mucosal ingrowth. Progressive tracheal collapse cranial or caudal to the original stent that causes clinical signs can be treated with placement of an additional stent or extraluminal ring placement for cervical collapse (**Fig. 6**).

Stent fractures occur with excessive cycling of the nitinol metal and are most likely to happen in oversized stents; excessive compression by incomplete opening decreases the stent's strength. Fractures tend to occur in the dorsal intrathoracic segment of the stent, because this is the area often oversized when the tracheal diameter is not uniform (**Fig. 7**). Fractures need to be differentiated from stent fraying, which

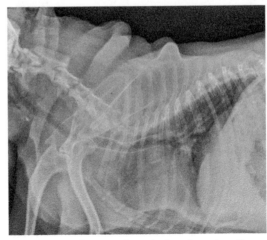

Fig. 7. Tracheal stent fracture in the intrathoracic dorsal stent wall.

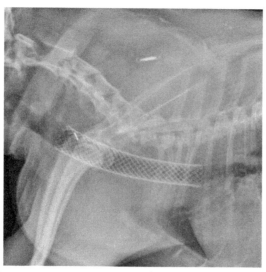

Fig. 8. Mild stent fraying at the cranial aspect of the stent. This patient had no clinical signs, and tracheal stent function was not impacted.

often occurs at the cranial aspect of the stent and is not problematic for stent function or patient comfort (**Fig. 8**). It is also important to understand differences in manufacturing, because Boston Scientific WallStents (Boston Scientific, Malborough, MA) are made of multiple woven wires and have free wire ends that are not fractures (**Fig. 9**). Mild fractures of the stent that do not affect its structural integrity may be closely monitored. Fractures that worsen coughing or cause weakening of the stent's ability to maintain a patent airway require placement of an additional stent within the original stent (**Fig. 10**).[34–36]

Inflammatory/granulomatous tissue formation in dogs with tracheal stents is poorly understood. Currently, it is thought to occur in patients with areas of poor mucosal ingrowth into the stent, resulting in mucous accumulation and chronic infections.[37,40] Limited experience with obstructive intraluminal granulomatous/inflammatory tissue has also shown promising response to immunosuppressive steroid therapy, culture-guided antibiotic therapy, and in some cases, repeat stenting (**Fig. 11**). More work

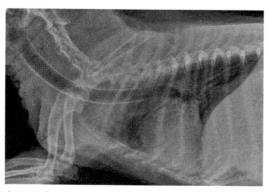

Fig. 9. Multiple end wires that are normal construction.

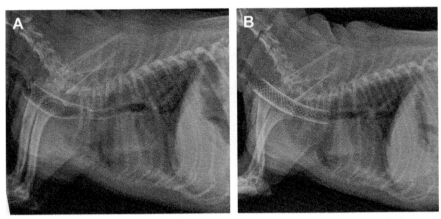

Fig. 10. Severe tracheal stent fracture that compromised stent function (A) and placement of a second stent within the first to support the fracture (B).

is needed to understand the cause of granulomatous/inflammatory tissue, role of infection, and optimal management strategies.

Even with the possible complications associated with tracheal stenting, it is still a viable method at relieving life-threatening airway obstructions and improving quality of life.[24,25,31,39]

BRONCHIAL STENTING

Collapse of the bronchi may occur in conjunction with tracheal collapse, secondary to compression from cardiomegaly, in association with brachycephalic airway disease, or as an isolated disease process.[7,8,13,19,28,40–44] In dogs with left atrial enlargement, collapse of the left mainstem bronchus alone has been reported.[45–47] In most of the other disease states, collapse is not localized to the mainstem bronchi only; the lobar bronchi are also affected. In cases where collapse is isolated to the mainstem bronchi only, bronchial stenting can be considered when bronchial compression is associated with clinical signs negatively affecting the patient's quality of life, particularly, paroxysms of coughing and resultant cyanosis and respiratory distress.[45] In a published case report of bronchial stenting in a dog, the pateint developed acute pulmonary edema after stent placement of unknown cause that required diuretic therapy and positive pressure ventilation. The dog survived for 102 days with self-limiting coughing

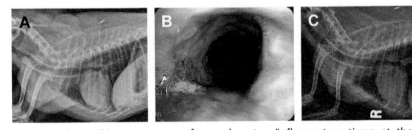

Fig. 11. Radiographic appearance of granulomatous/inflammatory tissue at the cranial aspect of a stent (A). Tracheoscopy demonstrating mucous accumulation and inflammatory tissue (B). Repeat thoracic radiographs 4 weeks after treatment with corticosteroids and culture-directed antibiotic therapy demonstrating resolution of the inflammatory tissue (C).

before succumbing to congestive heart failure.[45] In a recent abstract describing bronchial stenting in 17 dogs with severe collapse of the left cranial and caudal lobar bronchi, 16/17 dogs survived stent placement and 9/17 were alive at the time of submission of the abstract that spanned 2 years. However, only 2/17 dogs had no evidence of structural heart disease and 11/17 had no collapse of the tertiary bronchi. Therefore, the population of dogs with bronchial collapse/compression and concurrent cardiac disease likely needs to be compared separately to those dogs with diffuse collapse of the principle, lobar, and tertiary bronchi when deciding about candidacy and efficacy of bronchial stenting. Further investigation into this aspect of interventional management of airway collapse is needed.[47]

REFERENCES

1. White R, Williams JM. Tracheal collapse in the dog-is there really a role for surgery? A survey of 100 cases. J Small Anim Pract 1994;35(4):191–6.
2. Dallman MJ, McClure RC, Brown EM. Histochemical study of normal and collapsed tracheas in dogs. Am J Vet Res 1988;49(12):2117–25.
3. Mason RA, Johnson LR. Tracheal collapse. In: King LG, editor. Textbook of respiratory disease in dogs and cats. St Louis (MO): Saunders Publishing; 2004. p. 346–55.
4. Payne JD, Mehler SJ, Weisse C. Tracheal collapse. Compendium 2006;28(5): 373–83.
5. Sura PA, Krahwinkel DJ. Self-expanding nitinol stents for the treatment of tracheal collapse in dogs: 12 cases (2001–2004). J Am Vet Med Assoc 2008;232(2): 228–36.
6. Done SH, Drew RA. Observations on the pathology of tracheal collapse in dogs. J Sm Anim Pract 1976;17(12):783–91.
7. Johnson LR, Pollard RE. Tracheal collapse and bronchomalacia in dogs: 58 cases (7/2001-1/2008). J Vet Intern Med 2010;24(2):298–305.
8. Adamama-Moraitou KK, Pardali D, Dai MJ, et al. Canine bronchomalacia: a clinicopathological study of 18 cases diagnosed by endoscopy. Vet J 2012;191(2):261–6.
9. Bottero E, Bellino C, De Lorenzi D, et al. Clinical evaluation and endoscopic classification of bronchomalacia in dogs. J Vet Intern Med 2013;27(4):840–6.
10. Maggiore AD. Tracheal and airway collapse in dogs. Vet Clin North Am Small Anim Pract 2014;14(1):117–27.
11. Tanger CH, Hobson H. A retrospective study of 20 surgically managed cases of collapsed trachea. Vet Surg 1982;11(4):146–9.
12. Clarke DL. Upper airway disease. In: Silverstein DC, Hopper K, editors. Small animal critical care medicine. 2nd edition. St Louis (MO): Saunders Publishing; 2015. p. 92–104.
13. Macready DM, Johnson LR, Pollard RE. Fluoroscopic and radiographic evaluation of tracheal collapse in dogs: 62 cases (2001–2006). J Am Vet Med Assoc 2007;230(12):1870–6.
14. Nafe LA, Roberston ID, Hawkins EC. Cervical lung lobe herniation in dogs identified by fluoroscopy. Can Vet J 2013;54(10):955–9.
15. Rubin JA, Holt DE, Reetz JA, et al. Signalment, clinical presentation, concurrent diseases, and diagnostic findings in 28 dogs with dynamic pharyngeal collapse. J Vet Intern Med 2015;29(3):815–21.
16. Stadler K, Hartman S, Matheson J, et al. Computed tomography imaging of dogs with primary laryngeal or tracheal airway obstruction. Vet Radiol Ultrasound 2011; 52(4):377–84.

17. Scansen BA. Tracheal diameter and area: computed tomography versus fluoroscopy for stent sizing in 12 dogs with tracheal collapse. J Vet Intern Med 2014;(4): 1364.
18. Heyer CM, Nuesslein TG, Jung D, et al. Tracheobronchial anomalies and stenoses: detection with low-dose multidetector CT with virtual tracheobronchoscopy-comparison with flexible tracheobronchoscopy. Radiology 2007;242(2):542–9.
19. Johnson LR, Fales WH. Clinical and microbiologic findings in dogs with bronchoscopically diagnosed tracheal collapse: 37 cases (1990-1995). J Am Vet Med Assoc 2001;219(9):1247–50.
20. Johnson LR. Laryngeal structure and function in dogs with cough. J Am Vet Med Assoc 2016;249(2):195–201.
21. McKiernan BC, Smith AR, Kissil M. Bacterial isolates from the lower trachea of clinically healthy dogs. J Am Anim Hosp Assoc 1984;20:139–42.
22. Buback JL, Boothe HW, Hobson HP. Surgical treatment of tracheal collapse in dogs: 90 cases. J Am Vet Med Assoc 1996;208:380–4.
23. Clarke DL, Luskin A, Brown D. Endotracheal wash cytology and microbiologic results in dogs undergoing tracheal stenting: 34 cases (2011-2014). J Vet Emerg Crit Care 2015;25(S1):S3.
24. McGuire L, Winters C, Beal MW. Emergency tracheal stent placement for the relief of life-threatening airway obstruction in dogs with tracheal collapse. J Vet Emerg Crit Care 2013;23(S1):S9.
25. Beal MW. Tracheal stent placement for the emergency management of tracheal collapse in dogs. Top Companion Anim Med 2013;28(3):106–11.
26. Becker WM, Beal M, Stanley BJ, et al. Survival after surgery for tracheal collapse and the effect of intrathoracic collapse on survival. Vet Surg 2012;41(4):501–6.
27. Gellasch KL, Gomez TDC, McAnulty JF, et al. Use of intraluminal nitinol stents in the treatment of tracheal collapse in a dog. J Am Vet Med Assoc 2002;221(12): 1719–23.
28. Moritz A, Schneider M, Bauer N. Management of advanced tracheal collapse in dogs using intraluminal self-expanding biliary wallstents. J Vet Intern Med 2004; 18(1):31–42.
29. Sun F, Usón J, Ezquerra J, et al. Endotracheal stenting therapy in dogs with tracheal collapse. Vet J 2008;175(2):186–93.
30. Kim JY, Han HJ, Yun HY, et al. The safety and efficacy of a new self-expandable intratracheal nitinol stent for the tracheal collapse in dogs. J Vet Sci 2008;9(1):91–3.
31. Durant AM, Sura P, Rohrbach B, et al. Use of nitinol stents for end-stage tracheal collapse in dogs. Vet Surg 2012;41(7):807–17.
32. Culp WT, Weisse C, Cole SG, et al. Intraluminal tracheal stenting for treatment of tracheal narrowing in three cats. Vet Surg 2007;36(2):107–13.
33. Radlinsky MG, Fossum TW, Walker MA, et al. Evaluation of the Palmaz stent in the trachea and mainstem bronchi of normal dogs. Vet Surg 1997;26(2):99–107.
34. Mittleman E, Weisse C, Mehler SJ, et al. Fracture of an endoluminal nitinol stent used in the treatment of tracheal collapse in a dog. J Am Vet Med Assoc 2004; 225(8):1217–21, 1196.
35. Ouellet M, Dunn ME, Lussier B, et al. Noninvasive correction of a fractured endoluminal nitinol tracheal stent in a dog. J Am Anim Hosp Assoc 2006;42(6):467–71.
36. Woo HM, Kim MJ, Lee SG, et al. Intraluminal tracheal stent fracture in a Yorkshire terrier. Can Vet J 2007;48:1063–6.
37. Weisse CW. Intraluminal tracheal stenting. In: Weisse CW, Berent AC, editors. Veterinary image guided interventions. Ames (IA): Wiley Blackwell; 2015. p. 73–82.

38. Cleroux A, Brown D, Clarke DL. Evaluation of different endotracheal tube positions and peak airway pressures on maximal tracheal diameter measurements in dogs undergoing tracheal stenting. Veterinary Interventional Radiology & Interventional Endoscopy Society (VIRIES). Jackson Hole, WY, June 13–15, 2016.
39. Clarke DL, Tappin S, de Madron E, et al. Evaluation of a novel tracheal stent for the treatment of tracheal collapse in dogs. J Vet Intern Med 2014;(4):1364.
40. Weisse CW. Insights in tracheobronchial stenting and a theory of bronchial compression. J Small Anim Pract 2014;55(4):181–4.
41. Marolf A, Blaik M, Specht A. A retrospective study of the relationship between tracheal collapse and bronchiectasis in dogs. Vet Rad Ultrasound 2007;48(3): 199–203.
42. Clercx C, Peeters D, Snaps F, et al. Eosinophilic bronchopneumonopathy in dogs. J Vet Intern Med 2000;14:282–91.
43. De Lorenzi D, Bertoncello D, Drigo M. Bronchial abnormalities found in a consecutive series of 40 brachycephalic dogs. J Am Vet Med Assoc 2009;235:835–40.
44. Norris CR, Griffey SM, Samii VF, et al. Comparison of results of thoracic radiography, cytologic evaluation of bronchoalveolar lavage fluid, and histologic evaluation of lung specimens in dogs with respiratory tract disease: 16 cases (1996–2000). J Am Vet Med Assoc 2001;218:1456–61.
45. Dengate A, Culvenor JA, Graham K, et al. Bronchial stent placement in a dog with bronchomalacia and left atrial enlargement. J Small Anim Pract 2014;55:225–8.
46. Kramer G, McKiernan B, Burk R. Evaluation of bronchial collapse in dogs with chronic valvular heart disease. J Vet Intern Med 2008;22(3):757.
47. Kramer G, Ozer D, Williams B, et al. Bronchial stenting in dogs and development of a new bifurcated bronchial stent and delivery system. Abstract presented at Veterinary Interventional Radiology & Interventional Endoscopy Society (VIRIES) Meeting, Lisbon, Portugal, May 15–28, 2018.

Interventional Radiology Management of Vascular Malformations

Portosystemic Shunts and Vascular Fistulae/Malformations

William T.N. Culp, VMD*, Maureen A. Griffin, DVM

KEYWORDS

- Portosystemic shunt • Intrahepatic portosystemic shunt • Vascular malformation
- Arteriovenous malformation • Embolization

KEY POINTS

- Vascular malformations are uncommon in companion animals, although those affecting the liver occur with relative frequency.
- Diagnostic imaging is essential for thorough assessment of vascular malformations and to assist with treatment planning.
- Minimally invasive, image-guided techniques hold tremendous potential for the treatment of vascular malformations and early results are promising.

INTRODUCTION

Vascular malformations are abnormalities of the vascular system that are often classified based on their endothelial characteristics, such as arterial, venous, arteriovenous, capillary, lymphatic, and combined vascular malformations.[1] In companion animals, abnormal vascular connections involving the liver occur most readily, but these malformations can be diagnosed in any location. Portosystemic shunts (PSS) are the most common malformation described in veterinary patients, and much literature has focused on this topic. However, arteriovenous fistulae (AVF) and arteriovenous malformations (AVM) have also been reported multiple times. Although surgical treatment of PSS, AVF, and AVM can be pursued in many situations, other techniques are emerging as acceptable treatment options for these diseases. Interventional radiology (IR) techniques hold advantages over other treatment modalities because the

Department of Surgical and Radiological Sciences, School of Veterinary Medicine, University of California-Davis, One Shields Avenue, Davis, CA 95616, USA
* Corresponding author.
E-mail address: wculp@ucdavis.edu

Vet Clin Small Anim 48 (2018) 781–795
https://doi.org/10.1016/j.cvsm.2018.05.002
0195-5616/18/© 2018 Elsevier Inc. All rights reserved.

vetsmall.theclinics.com

abnormal vascular connections can be mapped and more specifically targeted, and patients can be treated in a less invasive fashion. The outcomes associated with IR treatments such as embolization are encouraging, although extensive evaluation is still needed.

ANATOMIC CONSIDERATIONS

Portosystemic shunts can be congenital or acquired secondary to chronic portal hypertension. Congenital PSS most commonly involve 1 (and rarely 2 or more) intrahepatic or extrahepatic vessels that act to provide direct communication between the portal venous circulation and systemic venous circulation (caudal vena cava or azygos vein), allowing portal blood to bypass the liver. Extrahepatic PSS connect the portal vein, left gastric vein, splenic vein, cranial or caudal mesenteric vein, or gastroduodenal vein to the caudal vena cava or azygos vein. Intrahepatic PSS connect portal vein branches to the systemic circulation via the hepatic veins or abdominal vena cava.[2] Left-sided intrahepatic PSS (often consistent with patent ductus venosus) arise from the left portal vein branch, course through the left liver lobes or papillary process of the caudate lobe, and drain into a venous ampulla at its confluence with the left phrenic vein and left hepatic vein (cranial to the liver) before draining into the caudal vena cava at the level of the diaphragm.[3] Central intrahepatic PSS course through the right medial or quadrate lobes, and right-sided intrahepatic PSS course through the right lateral lobe or caudate process of the caudate lobe before draining into the vena cava.[2]

In comparison to congenital PSS, acquired PSS vessels are typically multiple, tortuous, and extrahepatic. Commonly, these vessels link a portal tributary to a renal vein or the caudal vena cava in the region of the kidneys.[4,5] However, shunt vessels connecting the portal system to gonadal, internal thoracic, or other systemic venous vessels can also occur.

AVF and AVM occur rarely in veterinary patients and are typically congenital diseases associated with communications between multiple high-pressure arterial and low-pressure venous vessels within the liver.[6,7] The term "malformation" is now preferred over "fistula" to describe this condition in most situations because the majority of affected animals have multiple abnormal communications rather than a single communication. These malformations are most commonly present in the right or central divisional hepatic lobes. Typically a single lobe is affected, but 20% of dogs with hepatic AVM have 2 affected lobes.[6] They generally appear as large, tortuous vessels along the surface of the affected lobes, and multiple acquired extrahepatic PSS vessels may also be present secondary to portal hypertension. Although hepatic AVM are classically macroscopic in nature, microscopic hepatic AVM may be suspected in cases of young dogs with identical clinical signs, including portal hypertension and/or ascites, and histopathologic findings of hepatic AVM in which a macroscopic hepatic AVM is not identified.[8] Nonhepatic vascular malformations have been rarely described in companion animals with locations including the spinal cord,[9] gastrointestinal tract,[10] orbit,[11] ear,[12] and limbs.[13–17]

PHYSIOLOGY

The majority (66%–75%) of congenital single PSS are extrahepatic in dogs and cats.[18,19] Most extrahepatic PSS occur in small breed dogs, and most intrahepatic PSS occur in large breed dogs.[18] Epidemiologic factors including breed, sex, and country of origin have been reported to have significant association with the anatomic location of intrahepatic PSS in dogs.[20]

When the primary defect is a vascular anomaly that connects the portal venous system to the systemic venous system (such as congenital/single PSS), clinical manifestations are caused by diversion of portal blood flow away from the liver. This is due to portal venous pressure in the liver typically being greater than caudal vena cava pressure.[2] Bypassing portal blood flow deprives the liver of trophic factors and oxygen, resulting in poor hepatocyte growth and function.[2] Relative to extrahepatic PSS, intrahepatic PSS are typically associated with a larger volume of portal blood that is shunted to the systemic circulation, often resulting in the development of earlier and more severe clinical signs than patients with extrahepatic PSS.[21,22]

Most clinical signs of PSS in dogs and cats are associated with hepatic encephalopathy, a condition that incorporates a variety of neurologic abnormalities. The abnormal liver cannot appropriately filter, metabolize, or eliminate neurotoxic substances that are absorbed from the gastrointestinal tract and drain through the portal system. The result is that these toxic substances enter the systemic circulation through the portal-systemic shunt vessels, causing adverse effects on multiple organs, particularly the central nervous system. With loss of liver function, ammonia is not appropriately converted to urea and glutamine by the urea cycle and acts in an excitotoxic fashion by causing an increased release of glutamate.[23] Hepatic encephalopathy (HE) is a complex and poorly understood condition, with multiple additional neurotoxins likely associated with its pathogenesis. Another important clinical manifestation of hepatic disease/failure is disturbance of secondary hemostasis due to altered production of coagulation factors.

Acquired PSS occur secondary to increased portal pressures that result in the opening of vestigial fetal blood vessels. These opened vessels act as a "pop-off valve" to accommodate the increased hydrostatic pressure within the portal venous system. Hepatic fibrosis, portal vein hypoplasia with portal hypertension, and hepatic AVM are the most common causes of acquired PSS in veterinary patients.[5,6] In cases of hepatic AVM, a high-pressure system is created when a branch of the hepatic artery communicates directly with a vein (often portal) through multiple abnormal shunting vessels within the liver. This high-pressure system causes hepatofugal (away from the liver) blood flow and portal vein arterialization. For conditions associated with high portal pressure (including acquired PSS and hepatic AVM), portal hypertension results and multiple acquired extrahepatic PSS recannulate to decompress the portal system.[2] Additional clinical manifestations, aside from liver failure and HE, are often related to the underlying cause of portal hypertension, as well as the portal hypertension itself, which can cause ascites and gastrointestinal hemorrhage.[2]

AVF or AVM may be congenital and associated with failure of differentiation of embryonic structures into arteries and veins or acquired secondary to trauma, ischemia, and neoplasia.[24,25] Arteriovenous malformations are most frequently reported in extremities.[24] With AVM, blood preferentially flows from the high peripheral vascular resistance circuit (arterial) to the low peripheral vascular resistance circuit (venous), thereby bypassing peripheral capillary beds and tissue.[24] Cardiac output increases due to compensation for decreased arterial blood pressure and blood flow to tissues distal to the AVM.[24] This occurs via the baroreceptor reflex, constriction of blood reservoirs, increased heart rate, contractility, stroke volume, increased venous return, and activation of the sympathoadrenal and renin–angiotensin–aldosterone systems.[24,26] The venous system compensates via dilation to accommodate the increased circulating blood volume, causing further reduction of peripheral vascular resistance.[24] This process results in a persistent stimulus to increase the total circulating blood volume, resulting in overload of cardiac venous return, pulmonary hypertension, and high output cardiac failure.[24] Local changes also occur at the AVM site, including the development and dilation of collateral circulation, possible retrograde blood flow in the distal artery and peripheral venous vessels, and structural changes of the vasculature including arterialization and venization.[24] Tissue distal to the AVM can also be affected by the altered blood flow with resultant ischemia and organ dysfunction.

DIAGNOSTICS

Changes on complete blood count, biochemistry panel, and urinalysis can be consistent with a diagnosis of PSS and/or hepatic AVM, although these changes alone are not specific or diagnostic. Microcytosis has been reported with or without normochromic nonregenerative anemia in 60% to 72% of dogs and 30% of cats with PSS.[27,28] A definitive cause for this finding is not known, but possible causes include aberrant iron transport, reduced serum iron concentration, decreased total iron-binding capacity, and increased Kupffer cell iron storage.[27,28] Common biochemical abnormalities arise from abnormal liver function and reduced hepatic synthesis. These findings include hypoalbuminemia, decreased blood urea nitrogen (BUN) level, hypocholesterolemia, and hypoglycemia. Elevations in serum liver enzymes are typically mild to moderate. On urinalysis, more than 50% of affected animals are hyposthenuric or isosthenuric.[2,29] This can be attributed to a decreased medullary concentration gradient associated with reduced hepatic urea production as well as hepatic encephalopathy with possible psychogenic polydipsia. Ammonium biurate crystals and urolithiasis may also be noted.

Liver function testing is often done on patients with PSS and hepatic AVM. Similar to other blood and urine tests, abnormalities can be suggestive or consistent with these diseases but are not definitively diagnostic. Bile acid testing is typically performed on a fasted (12 hour) sample and 2 hours postprandial sample and can be affected by the production, excretion, and recirculation of bile acids.[30,31] Animals with PSS classically have a persistent increase in postprandial bile acid levels due to shunting of reabsorbed bile acids into systemic circulation.[31] Increases in postprandial bile acids alone or as a paired sample have been reported as 100% sensitive for PSS in dogs and cats.[30,31] Ammonia baseline levels can also be assessed. One report documented that when optimal normal cutoff values for ammonia (57 μmol/L in dogs and 94 μmol/L in cats) are used, the sensitivity and specificity of this test improves to 91% and 84% in dogs and 83% and 86% in cats, respectively.[23]

Coagulation abnormalities are also frequently detected in dogs with PSS, although spontaneous hemorrhage is rare in these animals.[32–34] Dogs with PSS typically have prolonged activated partial thromboplastin time (aPTT) and normal prothrombin time; possible causes for prolonged coagulation times include abnormal hepatic synthesis, qualitative anomalies, and impaired clearance of coagulation factors.[35,36] This prolongation in aPTT has not been associated with an increased intraoperative bleeding tendency in these dogs.[36]

Abdominal ultrasonography is the most common first-line imaging modality for diagnosis of PSS. Ultrasound is also helpful to detect radiolucent urinary calculi in affected animals with hepatic vascular anomalies.[37] Common ultrasonographic findings in animals with congenital PSS include an anomalous shunt vessel, subjectively small liver, renal enlargement, and a reduced number of hepatic and portal veins.[38] Activity of the patient during ultrasonography can interfere with the ability to find and accurately characterize a shunt vessel, such that sedation may be needed. Ultrasound has a reported sensitivity of 74% to 95% and specificity of 67% to 100% with regard to the detection of PSS.[25,37–40] The sensitivity for diagnosis of intrahepatic PSS is reportedly greater (95%–100%) than that for extrahepatic PSS due to the surrounding liver parenchyma and generally larger size of intrahepatic shunt vessels.[37] Studies have noted correct identification of the shunt vessel as intrahepatic or extrahepatic in 92% to 98% of cases.[37,38] Ultrasonographic findings with hepatic AVM include tortuous anechoic tubular structures adjacent to or within hepatic parenchyma.[41] Color-flow and pulse-wave Doppler can be used with ultrasonography to aid in identification of vascular anomalies. Portal flow velocity has been reported as increased or variable (relative to a normal value of 15 cm/s) in 53% of dogs with extrahepatic PSS and 92% of dogs with intrahepatic PSS.[2]

Fluoroscopy is a useful imaging modality to diagnose and characterize PSS and determine response to therapy. Fluoroscopy is essential for performing transvascular coil embolization or endovascular treatment of AVF/AVM.[42–46] Jejunal vein catheterization and portovenography have been described and recently compared with computed tomography (CT) angiography.[42] Intraoperative portovenography did not provide additional information relative to the CT but was useful in determining if the appropriate vessel had been attenuated at surgery and to evaluate for other shunting vessels.[42]

The use of scintigraphy has been described with radioactive tracers being delivered transcolonically[45,47–49] and transsplenically.[50,51] In a study of 16 dogs, 6 were noted to have abnormal shunt fractions as determined by transcolonic scintigraphy after cellophane banding. Transcolonic scintigraphy successfully identified continued shunting in those cases, with 3 dogs having incomplete shunt closure and 3 dogs developing multiple acquired PSS.[47] For ultrasound-guided transsplenic portal scintigraphy, the splenic parenchyma is injected with sodium pertechnetate Tc 99m, and scintigraphic images are obtained.[50,51] When comparing transsplenic portal scintigraphy with per-rectal portal scintigraphy, transsplenic scintigraphy was shown to be 100% sensitive and specific for PSS diagnosis and significantly more likely to determine the number and termination of the shunts due to the higher-quality nature of the studies.[51]

Several studies have described the use of CT in the diagnosis and assessment of PSS.[52–56] Dual-phase angiographic CT has been shown to provide sufficient vascular opacification with excellent definition of hepatic arteries and veins as well as portal tributaries and branches.[57] One study describing the use of CT for assessing extrahepatic PSS noted 6 general types of shunts: splenocaval, splenoazygos, splenophrenic, right gastric-caval, right gastric-caval with caudal shunt loop, and right gastric-azygos with caudal shunt loop.[55] When compared with ultrasonography, CT is significantly more sensitive (96% vs 68%) for PSS diagnosis and 5.5 times more likely to correctly identify PSS.[58]

While uncommonly used clinically, magnetic resonance angiography (MRA) has also been described in the diagnosis of PSS in dogs.[59–61] One study noted that excellent 3-dimensional anatomic detail was obtained with MRA.[59] In a separate study, MRA was shown to be highly specific for the diagnosis of PSS and sensitive for determining anatomic location of single PSS.[61]

Hepatic volume is a useful biomarker in the assessment of response to the treatment of PSS. The liver volume as normalized to body weight has been determined in normal dogs and found to be 24.5 ± 5.6 cm^3/kg.[62] Significant increase in liver volume has been documented after the treatment of both extrahepatic PSS and intrahepatic PSS.[45,49,62,63] In a study that evaluated hepatic volume prior to and after placement of ameroid constrictors around extrahepatic PSS vessels, the change in liver volume postoperatively was significantly associated with preoperative liver volume, and dogs with lower preoperative liver volumes had greater increases in the percentage of liver volume growth. In addition, after treatment, all liver volumes were in the normal or above normal range.[49] Similarly, in a separate study evaluating coil embolization as a treatment for intrahepatic PSS, liver volume significantly increased in dogs after coil embolization.[45]

SURGICAL TREATMENT

Many surgical treatment options for single congenital PSS have been reported and include partial or complete ligation and gradual attenuation via ameroid constrictors, cellophane bands, or hydraulic occluders.[64–71] Gradual attenuation is preferred over acute occlusion of shunt vessels to reduce the risk of postoperative complications. In general, it is recommended that congenital shunts be attenuated as close as possible to their insertion sites on the systemic vasculature in order to redirect blood flow from all tributaries of the shunt. If the terminus of an intrahepatic portacaval shunt is not visible, attenuation of the vessel supplying or draining the shunt can be performed.

Surgical treatment of hepatic AVM involves resection of the affected liver lobes. Temporary inflow of the celiac or hepatic artery and portal vein can be occluded via Rumel tourniquets with or without occlusion of the caudal vena cava cranial and caudal to the liver, and a jejunal or splenic catheter can be placed for measurement of portal pressures. The affected liver lobe is mobilized by transection of attached ligaments, and parenchyma of unaffected lobes is bluntly dissected away from the affected lobe. Lobectomy is performed via mass ligation of the hilus or following isolation and ligation of the portal vein and hepatic artery supplying the affected lobe. If possible, the nutrient artery, portal vein branch, and biliary duct to the affected lobe are isolated and double ligated with silk. The nutrient artery can be occluded temporarily initially to confirm that it is the source of the malformation via evidence of decreased portal pressure.[6]

Peripheral (nonhepatic) AVF/AVM can be treated with a combination of ligation and resection. In addition, AVF/AVM located in the distal limb may be amenable to removal via amputation. Surgical management of peripheral AVF/AVM is very challenging due to generalized vascular proliferation in the region of the AVF/AVM as well as tissue swelling and alteration of normal anatomy.

INTERVENTIONAL MANAGEMENT

The main application of IR in the treatment of PSS is for coil embolization of intrahepatic PSS. Traditional open surgical procedures used in the treatment of intrahepatic PSS are considered challenging because these types of shunts are often located in regions that are difficult to access and require dissection of liver parenchyma. It is generally considered ideal to attenuate a PSS as close to its insertion as possible because this decreases the chance of missing additional shunting vessels. Because intrahepatic PSS vessels often insert on the vena cava in a very cranial position, this further complicates surgical treatment. For these reasons, as well as the potential benefit of decreased pain and earlier recovery, a minimally invasive approach, percutaneous transvenous embolization (PTE), has been developed.

Prior to PTE, a contrast-enhanced CT needs to be performed. The CT scan is used to characterize shunt anatomy and the rest of the hepatic vasculature and to select a caudal vena cava stent size in each case. Multiple CT images are evaluated and the diameter of the caudal vena cava is measured in 2 perpendicular planes (**Fig. 1**). The average of the measurements is generated, and a stent that is approximately 20% greater in diameter is chosen.

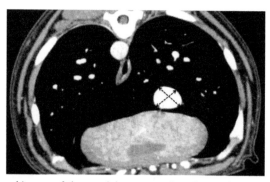

Fig. 1. Cross-sectional image of the caudal vena cava in a dog with an intrahepatic portosystemic shunt. The caudal vena cava is measured in perpendicular planes (*double headed arrows*) to determine the diameter of the stent that needs to be placed to cover the opening of the shunt insertion.

For the PTE procedure, the caudal venal cava and shunt are accessed percutaneously via the right jugular vein after placement of a vascular sheath, which permits catheter and wire passage while maintaining hemostasis without damage to the vessel. Under fluoroscopic guidance, coaxial passage of catheters and wires facilitates access into the PSS and then, if possible, into the portal vein. Once catheterization of the shunt/portal vein is confirmed with angiography, baseline portal and central venous pressures are obtained. A second guidewire and a marker catheter are advanced through the vascular access sheath into the caudal vena cava. A portogram and caudal vena cavogram are performed simultaneously to determine the location of the shunt ostium at the level of the vena cava. Based on the stent size determined on CT, a laser cut stent is chosen, placed over the guidewire, and deployed across the opening of the shunt ostium in the caudal vena cava. After stent placement, the shunt is accessed again across the interstices of the stent, and repeat measurements of the portal and caval pressures are performed to ensure stent placement did not excessively increase portal pressures. A second catheter is introduced into the shunt in the same fashion so that one catheter can be used to continuously measure portal pressures and the other can be used for deployment of thrombogenic coils to gradually occlude the shunt (**Fig. 2**). After delivery of each coil, the portal pressure is determined. A pressure gradient between the portal system and cranial vena cava of approximately 7 mm Hg and avoidance of portal pressures in excess of 18 to 20 mm Hg are considered therapeutic endpoints. A 7-Fr multilumen catheter is placed in the right jugular vein after removal of the vascular sheath to allow for vessel healing, and can be removed 1 to 2 days post-PTE.

The use of transvenous coil embolization was first documented in several case series.[72–76] Since that time, 2 major studies have been published that detail outcomes (both retrospectively and prospectively) in larger cohorts of dogs.[45,46] In the first study, 95 dogs with intrahepatic PSS had one treatment and 17% had multiple treatments.[46]

Intraprocedural complications were uncommon in that cohort of dogs and occurred in 14% of procedures. Major intraprocedural complications included substantial portal hypertension that was resolved following coil displacement (2 dogs) and severe acute gastrointestinal hemorrhage (1 dog), which accounted for the only intraprocedural death.[46] Life-threatening postprocedural complications included seizures/hepatic encephalopathy (6%), cardiac arrest (2%), hemorrhage from the jugular site requiring transfusion (2%), and one case each of pneumonia, suspected portal hypertension, and death of unknown cause.[46]

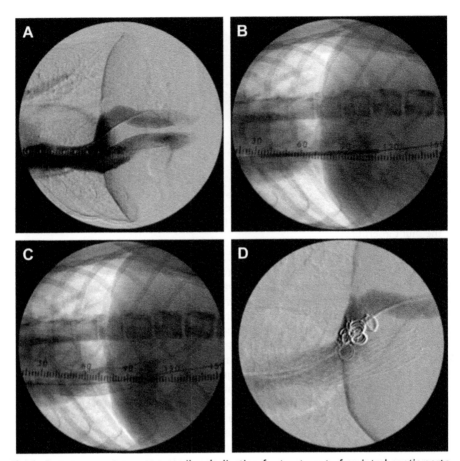

Fig. 2. Percutaneous transvenous coil embolization for treatment of an intrahepatic porto-systemic shunt (IHPSS) in a dog. (*A*) The dog is positioned in dorsal recumbency and a hooked catheter has been placed into the portal vein through the IHPSS and a marker catheter has been placed in the caudal vena cava. A dual angiogram has been performed to identify the involved blood vessels. (*B*) The guidewire and stent delivery system can be seen in the caudal vena cava. The stent guide can also be visualized in this image and is used to guide the location of stent deployment. (*C*) The stent has been deployed. Note the bulging of the stent in the region of the shunt ostium. (*D*) The vena cava stent and multiple coils have been placed. Two catheters have been placed through the interstices of the stent into the IHPSS. One catheter is positioned caudal to the coils to allow for an angiogram to be performed. The second catheter is used for coil delivery.

The median hospitalization time was 2 days with a range of 1 to 13 days.[46] Overall, outcome was considered excellent or fair in 66% and 15% of dogs, respectively, and median survival time after treatment was 2204 days. Several factors, including improvements in multiple laboratory values such as total solids concentration, bile acid concentration, albumin concentration, BUN concentration, and cholesterol concentration, were shown to be significantly associated with an excellent outcome.[46]

In another study, 25 dogs undergoing PTE were prospectively enrolled to evaluate changes in clinical signs, blood work, and diagnostic imaging after treatment.[45] All dogs in that study were medically managed before and after treatment with the same protocol. All dogs were discharged from the hospital after PTE. When comparing clinical signs before and after treatment, dogs were significantly less likely to have clinical signs such as vomiting, seizures, ataxia, head pressing, "star-gazing," lethargy, low energy level, unresponsiveness, polyuria, and polydipsia after treatment.[45] All affected blood work values improved by a minimum of 50% after treatment with significant improvements in mean corpuscular volume, BUN, total protein, albumin, cholesterol, alkaline phosphatase, and γ-glutamyl transferase. In addition, liver volumes increased significantly and hepatic arterial fraction decreased significantly posttreatment.[45] At recheck evaluation 3 months post-treatment, 92% of dogs were clinically normal off medications; 1 dog continued to demonstrate clinical signs related to the neurologic system and 1 dog had continued polyuria/polydipsia.[45]

In humans, the major treatment options for AVF/AVM are surgical resection, radiation therapy (generally stereotactic radiosurgery), and embolization.[77] For hepatic and peripheral AVF/AVM, transvascular techniques provide an attractive alternative to surgery due to the ability to target the fistula or nidus directly with a minimally invasive technique. In many cases, because of the advances in embolic agents, embolization is the treatment of choice for vascular anomalies in people.[1] The goal of treatment of AVM is to embolize the feeding arteries as close to the lesion as possible while completely eliminating the nidus. It is often desirable to leave the main access vessels patent to allow for future treatments.[78] The treatment of AVF/AVM in humans is often planned as a multiprocedure process as opposed to attempting to accomplish complete treatment in a single procedure[77]; this is more challenging in companion animals where the need for multiple anesthetic episodes and owner finances may preclude this approach. Regardless, when performing these procedures, nontarget embolization is a major complication and should be avoided.

Most AVF/AVM are approached from an artery that will allow the best access to the affected region. In the authors clinic, the surgical access to the femoral and carotid arteries is used most regularly. After placement of a vascular sheath with a hemostasis value, a series of diagnostic catheters can be used to select the major arterial supply of the AVF/AVM. Contrast angiography is performed periodically to delineate the blood supply to the abnormal vascular communications and nidus, which is often accessed with microwires and microcatheters.

Several embolic agents, including coils, particulate agents (eg, gelfoam, polyvinyl alcohol particles, spherical embolics), sclerosants, and liquid embolics have been investigated in the treatment of AVF and AVM.[79] A coil has been successfully used in treatment of a congenital AVF of the saphenous artery in a dog.[80] The delivery of particulate agents is generally used in the embolization of tumors as opposed to vascular malformations. In addition, with particulate agents, recanalization can occur, and if blood flow were reestablished, further therapy would be indicated.[81] Ultrasound can be used to target some anomalies with direct percutaneous access. For these cases, treatment can be performed with a sclerosing agent. This type of therapy should be reserved for low-flow lesions, because control of the sclerosing agent after direct injection is difficult and these sclerosants can cause systemic side effects when traveling beyond the lesion.[1] In addition, local extravasation of sclerosants can cause trauma to surrounding tissue.[1]

Liquid embolics that are used commonly in human patients include glue and ethylene vinyl alcohol copolymer dissolved in dimethyl sulfoxide (DMSO) (Onyx). Cyanoacrylate is the most common glue used and several variations have been developed. When cyanoacrylate comes into contact with an ionic milieu (eg, blood), polymerization occurs and results in embolization (**Fig. 3**).[77] Although many AVF/AVM can be successfully treated with cyanoacrylate, several challenges with the use of

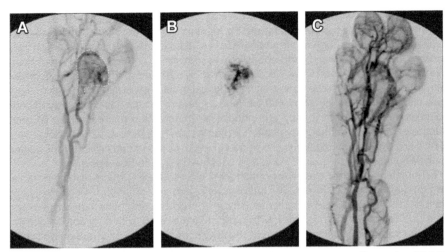

Fig. 3. Cyanoacrylate embolization of a metacarpal pad arteriovenous malformation (AVM). (*A*) In this preembolization image, an abnormally contrast-enhancing area can be noted in the metacarpal pad region (denoted with *white dashed line*). Note the poor perfusion present to the paw. (*B*) A microcatheter has been used to select the AVM nidus, and during this injection of contrast medium, only the AVM can be seen. The cyanoacrylate injection will be performed here. (*C*) After cyanoacrylate embolization, the AVM is not contrast-enhancing, and perfusion to the distal limb is markedly improved.

this product have been noted. Because rapid polymerization occurs when cyanoacrylate contacts blood, premature embolization may occur and subsequently prevent injection of cyanoacrylate into the AVF/AVM pedicle.[77] In addition, instruments that are used during these procedures can become embedded in the glue if not removed promptly after injection. Lastly, when embolization is performed with cyanoacrylate before surgical resection, a hard mass often forms and increases the challenge of removal.[77] Glue embolization of cranial abdominal and hepatic AVM have been described in dogs.[6,82,83] In a case series comparing surgical resection with glue embolization, the use of glue embolization was considered a good alternative to surgery because hepatic AVF-related death occurred less frequently in these patients.[6] In addition, of the 3 dogs that underwent glue embolization, all were still alive and had no clinical signs at a follow-up of 9 to 17 months.[6]

Onyx was originally manufactured for neurovascular indications, but over the last 10 years this product has been used in multiple other applications.[84] Onyx consists of ethylene vinyl alcohol copolymer dissolved in DMSO.[84] As Onyx is injected, an "outside-in" precipitation occurs in which an outer rim solidifies within the vessel and prevents the inner core from hardening; the result is that a semiliquid can continue to be injected down the center core as it is protected from polymerizing.[77,84] Onyx has several properties that make it attractive for use as a liquid embolic. First, Onyx is not a glue and therefore lacks adhesive properties.[77] This allows the Onyx to be injected without risk of adhesion between the microcatheter and the embolic. Second, the interaction of Onyx with the solvent, DMSO, prevents it from solidifying immediately on injection; essentially, the Onyx solidifies from the outer rim inside the vessel toward the center, thereby allowing for deeper penetration into the nidus when the operator is continuously injecting. Also, tantalum is added to the Onyx, which allows for excellent radio-opacity during injection. Lastly, because Onyx is not controlled by blood flow but instead by the injection of the operator, the delivery of Onyx is considered safe.[77] Recently, the use of Onyx to treat a peripheral AVM in the hindlimb of a dog was described.[13] In that case, the right hindlimb of a Tibetan Mastiff was swollen and the dog was minimally weight-bearing. After approaching the AVM via femoral artery access, Onyx was injected to fill the AVM nidus. The dog was discharged and no complications were noted. Within 2 weeks of the procedure, the swelling had markedly decreased and the dog was weight-bearing; at 4 weeks post-procedure, the circumference of the right hind paw was very similar to the normal left hind paw.[13] Onyx has also been used to treat a distal limb AVM in a cat and a brain AVM in a dog in the authors' clinic.

REFERENCES

1. Gloviczki P, Duncan A, Kalra M, et al. Vascular malformations: an update. Perspect Vasc Surg Endovasc Ther 2009;21:133–48.
2. Mathews KG, Bunch SK. Vascular liver diseases. In: Ettinger SJ, Feldman ED, editors. Textbook of veterinary internal medicine: diseases of the dog and cat. 6th edition. St Louis (MO): Saunders/Elsevier; 2005.
3. White RN, Burton CA. Anatomy of the patent ductus venosus in the dog. Vet Rec 2000;146:425–9.
4. Boothe HW, Howe LM, Edwards JF, et al. Multiple extrahepatic portosystemic shunts in dogs: 30 cases (1981-1993). J Am Vet Med Assoc 1996;208:1849–54.
5. Bunch SE, Johnson SE, Cullen JM. Idiopathic noncirrhotic portal hypertension in dogs: 33 cases (1982-1998). J Am Vet Med Assoc 2001;218:392–9.
6. Chanoit G, Kyles AE, Weisse C, et al. Surgical and interventional radiographic treatment of dogs with hepatic arteriovenous fistulae. Vet Surg 2007;36:199–209.
7. Legendre AM, Krahwinkel DJ, Carrig CB, et al. Ascites associated with intrahepatic arteriovenous fistula in a cat. J Am Vet Med Assoc 1976;168:589–91.
8. Schermerhorn T, Center SA, Dykes NL, et al. Suspected microscopic hepatic arteriovenous fistulae in a young dog. J Am Vet Med Assoc 1997;211:70–4.
9. Cordy DR. Vascular malformations and hemangiomas of the canine spinal cord. Vet Pathol 1979;16:275–82.
10. Gelens HC, Moreau RE, Stalis IH, et al. Arteriovenous fistula of the jejunum associated with gastrointestinal hemorrhage in a dog. J Am Vet Med Assoc 1993;202:1867–8.
11. Rubin LF, Patterson DF. Arteriovenous fistula of the orbit in a dog. Cornell Vet 1965;55:471–81.
12. Kealy JK, Lucey M, Rhodes WH. Arteriovenous fistula in the ear of a dog: a case report. J Small Anim Pract 1970;11:15–20.
13. Culp WT, Glaiberman CB, Pollard RE, et al. Use of ethylene-vinyl alcohol copolymer as a liquid embolic agent to treat a peripheral arteriovenous malformation in a dog. J Am Vet Med Assoc 2014;245:216–21.
14. Ettinger S, Campbell L, Suter PF, et al. Peripheral arteriovenous fistula in a dog. J Am Vet Med Assoc 1968;153:1055–8.
15. Furneaux RW, Pharr JW, McManus JL. Arterio-venous fistulation following dewclaw removal in a cat. J Am Anim Hosp Assoc 1974;10:569–73.
16. Jones DG, Allen WE, Webbon PM. Arteriovenous fistula in the metatarsal pad of a dog: a case report. J Small Anim Pract 1981;22:635–9.
17. Tobias KM, Cambridge A, Gavin P. Cyanoacrylate occlusion and resection of an arteriovenous fistula in a cat. J Am Vet Med Assoc 2001;219:785–8.
18. Winkler JT, Bohling MW, Tillson DM, et al. Portosystemic shunts: diagnosis, prognosis, and treatment of 64 cases (1993-2001). J Am Anim Hosp Assoc 2003;39:169–85.

19. Tivers M, Lipscomb V. Congenital portosystemic shunts in cats: investigation, diagnosis and stabilisation. J Feline Med Surg 2011;13:173–84.
20. Krotscheck U, Adin CA, Hunt GB, et al. Epidemiologic factors associated with the anatomic location of intrahepatic portosystemic shunts in dogs. Vet Surg 2007; 36:31–6.
21. Howe LM, Boothe HW. Diagnosis and treating portosystemic shunts in dogs and cats. Vet Med 2002;97:448.
22. Schermerhorn T, Center SA, Dykes NL, et al. Characterization of hepatoportal microvascular dysplasia in a kindred of cairn terriers. J Vet Intern Med 1996; 10:219–30.
23. Ruland K, Fischer A, Hartmann K. Sensitivity and specificity of fasting ammonia and serum bile acids in the diagnosis of portosystemic shunts in dogs and cats. Vet Clin Pathol 2010;39:57–64.
24. Hosgood G. Arteriovenous fistulas: pathophysiology, diagnosis, and treatment. Compendium 1989;11:625–36.
25. Lamb CR, White RN. Morphology of congenital intrahepatic portacaval shunts in dogs and cats. Vet Rec 1998;142:55–60.
26. Nakano J, DeSchryver C. Effects of arteriovenous fistula on systemic and pulmonary circulations. Am J Physiol 1964;207:1319–24.
27. Bunch SE, Jordan HL, Sellon RK, et al. Characterization of iron status in young dogs with portosystemic shunt. Am J Vet Res 1995;56:853–8.
28. Simpson KW, Meyer DJ, Boswood A, et al. Iron status and erythrocyte volume in dogs with congenital portosystemic vascular anomalies. J Vet Intern Med 1997; 11:14–9.
29. Broome CJ, Walsh VP, Braddock JA. Congenital portosystemic shunts in dogs and cats. N Z Vet J 2004;52:154–62.
30. Center SA, Baldwin BH, Erb HN, et al. Bile acid concentrations in the diagnosis of hepatobiliary disease in the dog. J Am Vet Med Assoc 1985;187:935–40.
31. Center SA, Erb HN, Joseph SA. Measurement of serum bile acids concentrations for diagnosis of hepatobiliary disease in cats. J Am Vet Med Assoc 1995;207: 1048–54.
32. Badylak SF, Dodds WJ, van Vleet JF. Plasma coagulation factor abnormalities in dogs with naturally occurring hepatic disease. Am J Vet Res 1983;44:2336.
33. Kummeling A, Teske E, Tothuizen J, et al. Coagulation profiles in dogs with congenital portosystemic shunts before and after surgical attenuation. J Vet Intern Med 2006;20:1319–26.
34. Papazoglou LG, Monnet E, Seim HB. Survival and prognostic indicators for dogs with intrahepatic portosystemic shunts: 32 cases (1990–2000). Vet Surg 2002;31: 561–70.
35. Kummeling A, Teske E, Rothuizen J, et al. Coagulation profiles in dogs with congenital portosystemic shunts before and after surgical attenuation. J Vet Intern Med 2006;20:1319–26.
36. Niles JD, Williams JM, Cripps PJ. Hemostatic profiles in 39 dogs with congenital portosystemic shunts. Vet Surg 2001;30:97–104.
37. Lamb CR, Forster-van Hijfte MA, White RN, et al. Ultrasonographic diagnosis of congenital portosystemic shunt in 14 cats. J Small Anim Pract 1996;37: 205–9.
38. d'Anjou MA, Penninck D, Cornejo L, et al. Ultrasonographic diagnosis of portosystemic shunting in dogs and cats. Vet Radiol Ultrasound 2004;45:424–37.
39. Tiemessen I, Rothuizen J, Voorhout G. Ultrasonography in the diagnosis of congenital portosystemic shunts in dogs. Vet Q 1995;17:50–3.

40. Holt DE, Schelling CG, Saunders HM, et al. Correlation of ultrasonographic findings with surgical, portographic, and necropsy findings in dogs and cats with portosystemic shunts: 63 cases (1987-1993). J Am Vet Med Assoc 1995;207:1190–3.
41. Bailey MQ, Willard MD, McLoughlin MA, et al. Ultrasonographic findings associated with congenital hepatic arteriovenous fistula in three dogs. J Am Vet Med Assoc 1988;192:1099–101.
42. Parry AT, White RN. Comparison of computed tomographic angiography and intraoperative mesenteric portovenography for extrahepatic portosystemic shunts. J Small Anim Pract 2017;58:49–55.
43. White RN, Parry AT. Morphology of congenital portosystemic shunts emanating from the left gastric vein in dogs and cats. J Small Anim Pract 2013;54:459–67.
44. White RN, Macdonald NJ, Burton CA. Use of intraoperative mesenteric portovenography in congenital portosystemic shunt surgery. Vet Radiol Ultrasound 2003; 44:514–21.
45. Culp WTN, Zwingenberger AL, Giuffrida MA, et al. Prospective evaluation of outcome of dogs with intrahepatic portosystemic shunts treated via percutaneous transvenous coil embolization. Vet Surg 2018;47:74–85.
46. Weisse C, Berent AC, Todd K, et al. Endovascular evaluation and treatment of intrahepatic portosystemic shunts in dogs: 100 cases (2001-2011). J Am Vet Med Assoc 2014;244:78–94.
47. Landon BP, Abraham LA, Charles JA. Use of transcolonic portal scintigraphy to evaluate efficacy of cellophane banding of congenital extrahepatic portosystemic shunts in 16 dogs. Aust Vet J 2008;86:169–79.
48. Samii VF, Kyles AE, Long CD, et al. Evaluation of interoperator variance in shunt fraction calculation after transcolonic scintigraphy for diagnosis of portosystemic shunts in dogs and cats. J Am Vet Med Assoc 2001;218:1116–9.
49. Zwingenberger AL, Daniel L, Steffey MA, et al. Correlation between liver volume, portal vascular anatomy, and hepatic perfusion in dogs with congenital portosystemic shunt before and after placement of ameroid constrictors. Vet Surg 2014; 43(8):926–34.
50. Morandi F, Cole RC, Tobias KM, et al. Use of 99mTCO4(-) trans-splenic portal scintigraphy for diagnosis of portosystemic shunts in 28 dogs. Vet Radiol Ultrasound 2005;46:153–61.
51. Sura PA, Tobias KM, Morandi F, et al. Comparison of 99mTcO4(-) trans-splenic portal scintigraphy with per-rectal portal scintigraphy for diagnosis of portosystemic shunts in dogs. Vet Surg 2007;36:654–60.
52. Frank P, Mahaffey M, Egger C, et al. Helical computed tomographic portography in ten normal dogs and ten dogs with a portosystemic shunt. Vet Radiol Ultrasound 2003;44:392–400.
53. Fukushima K, Kanemoto H, Ohno K, et al. Computed tomographic morphology and clinical features of extrahepatic portosystemic shunts in 172 dogs in Japan. Vet J 2014;199:376–81.
54. Hunt GB, Culp WT, Mayhew KN, et al. Evaluation of in vivo behavior of ameroid ring constrictors in dogs with congenital extrahepatic portosystemic shunts using computed tomography. Vet Surg 2014;43(7):834–42.
55. Nelson NC, Nelson LL. Anatomy of extrahepatic portosystemic shunts in dogs as determined by computed tomography angiography. Vet Radiol Ultrasound 2011; 52:498–506.
56. Zwingenberger AL, Schwarz T, Saunders HM. Helical computed tomographic angiography of canine portosystemic shunts. Vet Radiol Ultrasound 2005;46: 27–32.

57. Zwingenberger AL, Schwarz T. Dual-phase CT angiography of the normal canine portal and hepatic vasculature. Vet Radiol Ultrasound 2004;45:117–24.

58. Kim SE, Giglio RF, Reese DJ, et al. Comparison of computed tomographic angiography and ultrasonography for the detection and characterization of portosystemic shunts in dogs. Vet Radiol Ultrasound 2013;54:569–74.

59. Bruehschwein A, Foltin I, Flatz K, et al. Contrast-enhanced magnetic resonance angiography for diagnosis of portosystemic shunts in 10 dogs. Vet Radiol Ultrasound 2010;51:116–21.

60. Mai W, Weisse C. Contrast-enhanced portal magnetic resonance angiography in dogs with suspected congenital portal vascular anomalies. Vet Radiol Ultrasound 2011;52:284–8.

61. Seguin B, Tobias KM, Gavin PR, et al. Use of magnetic resonance angiography for diagnosis of portosystemic shunts in dogs. Vet Radiol Ultrasound 1999;40:251–8.

62. Stieger SM, Zwingenberger A, Pollard RE, et al. Hepatic volume estimation using quantitative computed tomography in dogs with portosystemic shunts. Vet Radiol Ultrasound 2007;48:409–13.

63. Kummeling A, Vrakking DJ, Rothuizen J, et al. Hepatic volume measurements in dogs with extrahepatic congenital portosystemic shunts before and after surgical attenuation. J Vet Intern Med 2010;24:114–9.

64. Hunt GB. Effect of breed on anatomy of portosystemic shunts resulting from congenital diseases in dogs and cats: a review of 242 cases. Aust Vet J 2004;82:746–9.

65. Kummeling A, Van Sluijs FJ, Rothuizen J. Prognostic implications of the degree of shunt narrowing and of the portal vein diameter in dogs with congenital portosystemic shunts. Vet Surg 2004;33:17–24.

66. Adin CA, Sereda CW, Thompson MS, et al. Outcome associated with use of a percutaneously controlled hydraulic occluder for treatment of dogs with intrahepatic portosystemic shunts. J Am Vet Med Assoc 2006;229:1749–55.

67. Frankel D, Seim H, MacPhail C, et al. Evaluation of cellophane banding with and without intraoperative attenuation for treatment of congenital extrahepatic portosystemic shunts in dogs. J Am Vet Med Assoc 2006;228:1355–60.

68. Lipscomb VJ, Jones HJ, Brockman DJ. Complications and long-term outcomes of the ligation of congenital portosystemic shunts in 49 cats. Vet Rec 2007;160:465–70.

69. Mehl ML, Kyles AE, Hardie EM, et al. Evaluation of ameroid ring constrictors for treatment for single extrahepatic portosystemic shunts in dogs: 168 cases (1995-2001). J Am Vet Med Assoc 2005;226:2020–30.

70. Sereda CW, Adin CA. Methods of gradual vascular occlusion and their applications in treatment of congenital portosystemic shunts in dogs: a review. Vet Surg 2005;34:83–91.

71. Tobias KM, Rohrbach BW. Association of breed with the diagnosis of congenital portosystemic shunts in dogs: 2,400 cases (1980-2002). J Am Vet Med Assoc 2003;223:1636–9.

72. Asano K, Watari T, Kuwabara M, et al. Successful treatment by percutaneous transvenous coil embolization in a small-breed dog with intrahepatic portosystemic shunt. J Vet Med Sci 2003;65:1269–72.

73. Bussadori R, Bussadori C, Millan L, et al. Transvenous coil embolisation for the treatment of single congenital portosystemic shunts in six dogs. Vet J 2008;176:221–6.

74. Gonzalo-Orden JM, Altonaga JR, Costilla S, et al. Transvenous coil embolization of an intrahepatic portosystemic shunt in a dog. Vet Radiol Ultrasound 2000;41: 516–8.

75. Leveille R, Johnson SE, Birchard SJ. Transvenous coil embolization of portosystemic shunt in dogs. Vet Radiol Ultrasound 2003;44:32–6.

76. Leveille R, Pibarot P, Soulez G, et al. Transvenous coil embolization of an extrahepatic portosystemic shunt in a dog: a naturally occurring model of portosystemic malformations in humans. Pediatr Radiol 2000;30:607–9.

77. Ayad M, Eskioglu E, Mericle RA. Onyx: a unique neuroembolic agent. Expert Rev Med Devices 2006;3:705–15.

78. Allison DJ, Kennedy A. ABC of vascular diseases. Peripheral arteriovenous malformations. BMJ 1991;303:1191–4.

79. Legiehn GM, Heran MK. Classification, diagnosis, and interventional radiologic management of vascular malformations. Orthop Clin North Am 2006;37:435–74.

80. Saunders AB, Fabrick C, Achen SE, et al. Coil embolization of a congenital arteriovenous fistula of the saphenous artery in a dog. J Vet Intern Med 2009;23: 662–4.

81. Dickey KW, Pollak JS, Meier GH 3rd, et al. Management of large high-flow arteriovenous malformations of the shoulder and upper extremity with transcatheter embolotherapy. J Vasc Interv Radiol 1995;6:765–73.

82. Case JB, Boston SE, Porter EP, et al. Endovascular treatment of a high-flow hepatic arteriovenous malformation with secondary portal hypertension in a dog. J Am Vet Med Assoc 2017;251:824–8.

83. Eason BD, Hogan DF, Lim C, et al. Use of n-butyl cyanoacrylate to reduce left to right shunting of an abdominal arteriovenous malformation in a dog. J Vet Cardiol 2017;19:396–403.

84. Kilani MS, Izaaryne J, Cohen F, et al. Ethylene vinyl alcohol copolymer (Onyx) in peripheral interventional radiology: indications, advantages and limitations. Diagn Interv Imaging 2015;95:319–26.

Cardiac Interventions in Small Animals
Areas of Uncertainty

Brian A. Scansen, DVM, MS

KEYWORDS

- Canine • Feline • Veterinary • Stent • Balloon • Cardiac catheterization

KEY POINTS

- Advanced therapies, such as high-pressure balloon dilation, cutting or scoring balloon dilation, or stent implantation, may play a role in interventional therapies for pulmonary valve stenosis.
- Cutting or high-pressure balloon dilation may play a role in palliating subaortic or valvar aortic stenosis in dogs.
- Transvenous coil embolization using controlled delivery coils may offer interventional closure to animals too small for transarterial device occlusion of patent ductus arteriosus.
- In rare cases of cyanotic heart disease, ductal stenting may improve pulmonary blood flow and provide a minimally invasive alternative to surgical placement of an aortopulmonary shunt.
- Strategies to avoid surgical exposure of blood vessels for vascular access in dogs include ultrasound guidance and vascular closure devices.

INTRODUCTION

The number of diseases afflicting dogs and cats that are amenable to treatment by a minimally invasive, transcatheter approach continues to expand. Cardiac interventions that are commonly performed in small animals include balloon dilation of congenitally stenotic valves,[1,2] coil or device occlusion of anomalous vessels,[3–5] extraction of parasites or foreign material from the heart and vasculature,[6] and pacing for symptomatic bradycardia.[7–9] Rarely, device closure of septal defects, intracardiac stents, and transcatheter valve implantation are also performed in veterinary patients. Cardiac interventions have been described and performed in animals for more than 30 years.[10,11] In that time, broad

Disclosure Statement: The author has received speaking fees, travel reimbursement, or products at no cost for development/preclinical evaluation from the following companies relevant to this publication: Infiniti Medical, LLC; Avalon Medical, Inc; and Dextronix, Inc.
Cardiology and Cardiac Surgery, Department of Clinical Sciences, Colorado State University, Campus Delivery 1678, Fort Collins, CO 80523, USA
E-mail address: Brian.Scansen@colostate.edu

advancements in both equipment and technique have occurred in the human medical arena that have been variably adopted by the veterinary community. Although interventional procedures are now standard of care for animals with some forms of heart disease, there remain areas of uncertainty in optimal technique, preferred candidates for intervention, and expected outcome. This article is not intended to provide definitive answers to these uncertainties, but rather to highlight issues currently in need of study and to offer the author's opinion and experience. Specific items to be addressed include variants of pulmonary valve anatomy and alternatives to conventional balloon dilation for pulmonary valve stenosis (PS), patient selection for cutting or high-pressure balloon dilation of aortic valvar or subaortic stenosis (SAS), occlusion of patent ductus arteriosus (PDA) in small dogs, ductal stenting in conditions with reduced pulmonary flow, and alternative considerations for vascular access and closure.

PULMONARY VALVE STENOSIS

Congenital PS was originally reported as the third most commonly diagnosed congenital heart defect of dogs in North America,[12] although more recent reports suggest it is the most common canine congenital heart defect.[13,14] Without therapy, dogs with PS are at risk for symptoms including exercise intolerance, syncope, sudden cardiac death, congestive heart failure, and cyanosis from a right-to-left shunt.[15,16]

There is evidence that balloon pulmonary valvuloplasty (BPV) improves the outcome of human and canine patients with PS, reducing clinical signs and improving survival.[15,17,18] The procedure is now routinely performed in clinical canine practice with low morbidity and mortality for those animals with a severe gradient or the presence of clinical signs referable to their disease. For a stepwise description of this interventional procedure, please see other resources.[1,19]

Is the Correct Term Pulmonary Valve Stenosis or Pulmonic Stenosis?

Veterinary cardiologists differ in terminology when referring to the semilunar valve that separates the right ventricle from the pulmonary trunk. The veterinary cardiology literature often ascribes the term pulmonic valve to describe this structure, yet the *Nomina Anatomica Veterinaria* term for this valve is *valva trunci pulmonalis*, which when anglicized becomes the valve of the pulmonary trunk.[20] In *Miller's Anatomy of the Dog*, the anatomic term given is pulmonary valve.[21] One of the first published descriptions of the disease in humans was provided by Arthur Keith[22] in the Hunterian Lectures on the Malformations of the Heart, in which the term pulmonary stenosis was used. The International Nomenclature and Database Conference for Pediatric Cardiac Surgery defines the disease as pulmonary stenosis with intact ventricular septum, and then subdivides these into subvalvar, valvar, and supravalvar sites of stenosis.[23] Within the veterinary literature, David Detweiler's article on heart disease in the second edition of *Canine Medicine* describes the condition as common in the dog and uses the nomenclature pulmonary stenosis.[24] Last, in the seminal description of the disease in the beagle dog by Don Patterson and colleagues,[25] based on the breeding colony at the University of Pennsylvania, both pulmonary stenosis and dysplasia of the pulmonary valve are the terms ascribed to the condition. It is the author's opinion that the correct term for this condition in animals is pulmonary stenosis and, for most cases in small animals, the site of obstruction is at the pulmonary valve.

Which Valve Morphology Is Amenable to Balloon Pulmonary Valvuloplasty?

PS in dogs has variable features, several of which impact the potential for a successful intervention. Transthoracic echocardiography with Doppler is the current standard of care in veterinary cardiology for evaluation of pulmonary valve morphology, annular size, and severity of stenosis. In humans, the most common form of the disease is the domed or typical form.[26] In domed PS, there is incomplete separation of the leaflets secondary to fusion along the valve commissures, systolic bowing into the pulmonary trunk, and poststenotic dilation of the pulmonary trunk itself. Dysplastic PS in the human is described as thickened leaflets with limited mobility and variable commissural fusion.[26] Other forms of pulmonary stenosis include infundibular (subvalvar) and supravalvar pulmonary stenosis.

Patterson and colleagues[25] work with the beagle colony described valve thickening, valve hypoplasia, and valve fusion; as such, they used the term pulmonary valve dysplasia broadly to describe these lesions. In more recent work, Bussadori and colleagues[27] categorized 2 forms of canine PS: type A, in which there was minimal leaflet thickening, fused commissures with a central orifice, systolic doming, an aortic/pulmonary annulus ratio less than 1.2, and poststenotic dilation of the pulmonary trunk; and type B, in which there was marked leaflet thickening, hypoplasia of the pulmonary annulus with an aortic/pulmonary annulus ratio greater than 1.2, severe infundibular hypertrophy, and rare or minimal poststenotic dilation of the pulmonary trunk. Using this classification, Bussadori and colleagues[27] showed that outcomes were worse for dogs with type B morphology. A recent large retrospective review of congenital heart disease used similar classification for canine PS, based on the relative diameters of the pulmonary valve annulus compared with the aortic valve annulus.[14] The author does not believe that canine PS fits easily into binary categories. Rather, valve thickening, valve fusion, annular hypoplasia, and poststenotic dilation each exist within a continuum in canine PS such that some dogs are affected primarily with fusion and systolic doming of the valve, others have thick leaflets with a hypoplastic annulus, and still others have features of each (**Fig. 1**).

Although the optimal categorization scheme for canine PS is undefined, it is useful to specifically evaluate the features described previously in each case and determine how much of the stenosis appears secondary to valve fusion, valve thickening, and/or annular hypoplasia. Certainly, cases that display more features consistent with "typical" or "type A" PS have a better response to BPV than those cases that have features most consistent with a "dysplastic" or "type B" PS. It is not uncommon, however, to treat dogs that have thick leaflets with an uncertain degree of valve fusion and a normal to small annulus that still have good results after BPV. Although preoperative evaluation is useful and may help predict the success of BPV; in the author's experience, definitive arbitration of what will be a successful versus an unsuccessful BPV is not yet possible by current methods of echocardiographic assessment.

The term supravalvar stenosis has been used to describe dogs with PS and obstructive fibrous tissue at the tip of the valve leaflets or at the sinotubular junction. In the author's opinion, this remains within the spectrum of PS, as the sinotubular junction belongs to the valve apparatus. True supravalvar pulmonary stenosis is rare in the dog, is perhaps better termed pulmonary artery stenosis,[14] and is defined as a narrowing anatomically distant from the sinotubular junction. Many cases of canine PS, perhaps even most, have fibrous adhesions between the leaflet tips and the sinotubular junction, and these typically open well with BPV (**Fig. 2**).

Should All Dogs Receive Beta-Blockade Before Balloon Pulmonary Valvuloplasty?

The decision to medicate a dog with beta-blockers before BPV is made on a case-by-case basis. The author believes that most dogs with severe stenosis will benefit from starting atenolol for 2 to 4 weeks before the BPV procedure. Beta-blockade decreases the force of right ventricular contraction, slows heart rate, and reduces myocardial

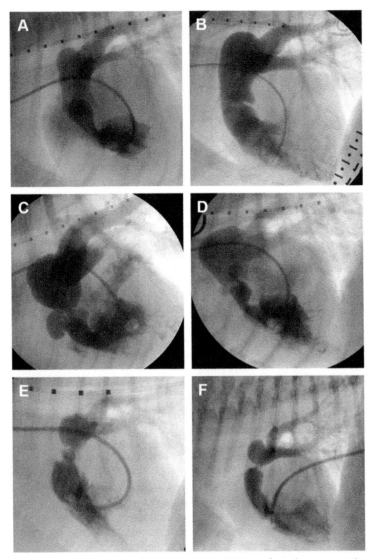

Fig. 1. The spectrum of valvar morphology in canine PS is very broad, encompassing variable degrees of valvar fusion, valvar thickening, obstructive fibrous tissue, and annular hypoplasia. Some representative right ventriculograms from dogs with severe PS are shown, demonstrating a normal-size pulmonary valve annulus with thin, fused valves (*A*); a normal-size pulmonary valve annulus with mild valvar thickening and fusion (*B*); a normal-size pulmonary valve annulus with valvar thickening, fibrous obstruction at the sinotubular junction, and an aneurysmal cranial sinus (*C*); moderate annular hypoplasia with severe valve thickening (*D*); annular hypoplasia with valvar fusion and fibrous obstruction at the sinotubular junction (*E*); and severe annular hypoplasia with valvar thickening and fibrous obstruction (*F*). Note that in all cases, moderate to severe poststenotic dilation of the pulmonary trunk is apparent.

oxygen consumption. These effects may improve anesthetic stability, reduce the dynamic component of stenosis that develops due to severe infundibular hypertrophy, and provide a slower heart rate during the procedure, which facilitates accurate balloon placement. A dose of 0.5 mg/kg by mouth every 12 hours is typically started,

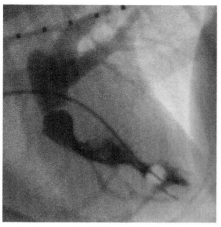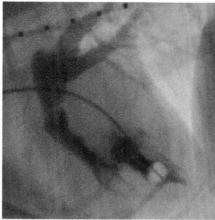

Fig. 2. Systolic (*left*) and diastolic (*right*) frames during right ventriculography in a dog with PS. In addition to valvar fusion, the leaflets demonstrate fusion to aberrant fibrous tissue at the sinotubular junction. This is observed commonly in canine PS and also can be seen in (*B–E*) of **Fig. 1** and the upper left panel of **Fig. 3**.

increasing to 1.0 to 1.5 mg/kg by mouth every 12 hours over the following 1 to 2 weeks. Dogs with severe dynamic obstruction below the valve as a result of muscular hypertrophy often benefit from even higher doses of atenolol (up to 2 or 3 mg/kg by mouth every 12 hours). Postponing BPV for 2 to 4 weeks can be particularly beneficial in very young dogs, as it allows for somatic growth that will reduce anesthetic risk and increase the likelihood of successful BPV. Although dogs weighing less than 1 kg can undergo BPV, their small vasculature and reduced right ventricular lumen greatly complicate the passage of wires and catheters necessary for a successful procedure.

What Can Be Done for Dogs that Do Not Improve with Conventional Balloon Pulmonary Valvuloplasty?

The original balloon dilation catheters were designed for vascular lesions, not valves. They were large and of limited use in small patients. Balloons specifically designed for BPV, having low profile, rapid inflation/deflation characteristics, and good trackability through the right heart, are now available on the human market and work well for dogs; however, most human cases are typical PS that respond well to low-pressure balloon dilation. In humans, the dysplastic form of PS, which is often comparable to many if not most cases of canine PS, has less successful results following BPV as compared with the domed form of PS.[28] Various strategies have been used to improve the success of transcatheter interventions in dogs that do not respond to conventional BPV, including the use of high-pressure balloons, cutting balloon dilation catheters, and intracardiac stents.

High-pressure balloon dilation catheters, which generate high internal pressure to effect greater radial force than conventional balloons, are commercially available in sizes useful for BPV. High-pressure BPV, arbitrarily defined as balloon inflation pressures exceeding 8 atm, has been advocated for resistant PS in children with pressure gradient reduction noted even in patients who had previously failed conventional BPV.[28] Reports of high-pressure BPV in dogs have been published,[29,30] which anecdotally suggest good to superior outcomes can be achieved even in dysplastic or type B cases. Currently, the author selects high-pressure balloon dilation catheters for nearly all cases of canine PS unless limited by size of vascular access, for very small dogs in which stiffer high-pressure balloon dilation catheters are more problematic to navigate through the right ventricle, or if valve morphology is that of pure valve fusion with no/minimal thickening or annular hypoplasia. Sizing of high-pressure balloon dilation catheters is comparable to conventional BPV; a balloon-to-annulus ratio of 1.3 to 1.5 is selected (**Fig. 3**). Superstiff guidewires are advised for high-pressure BPV, as the stiff catheter shaft can distort soft or standard stiffness guidewires and risk damage to the pulmonary trunk or a suboptimal inflation. Prospective studies are needed to validate this approach.

If higher inflation pressure can result in improved dilation of resistant stenoses, the ability to cut or score resistant tissue before dilation may further improve efficacy of balloon dilation. The use of transcatheter cutting balloon technology to treat PS was first attempted more than 20 years ago when a double-blade balloon was used to open a stenotic pulmonary valve in a dog model, followed by its use in 3 children.[31] Specialized balloon dilation catheters with cutting blades or scoring wires are now available, which expose microblades or a nitinol scoring wire arranged helically around the balloon during inflation to cut/score the lesion. A small case series described the use of cutting balloons in 4 children with variable degrees of valvar PS and infundibular narrowing/hypertrophy in the setting of tetralogy of Fallot.[32] These investigators found the technique safe and effective, resulting in significant improvement in clinical status and obviating the need for prompt surgical intervention. More recently, 5 children with

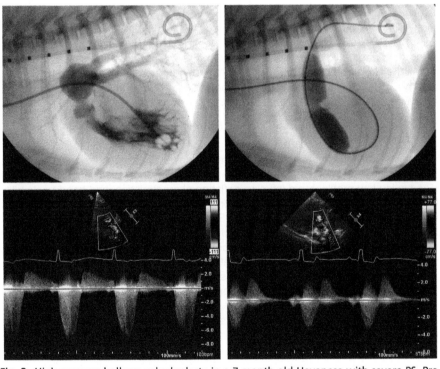

Fig. 3. High-pressure balloon valvuloplasty in a 7-month-old Havanese with severe PS. Preoperative transpulmonary gradient was approximately 155 mm Hg with both a fixed and dynamic spectral Doppler profile (*lower left*) and the right ventriculogram demonstrated valvar fusion with fibrous adhesions to the sinotubular junction (*upper left*). High-pressure balloon inflation was performed to 9 atm pressure (*upper right*) and resulted in a 71% reduction in transpulmonary gradient to ~45 mm Hg (*lower right*).

dysplastic PS who failed to respond to standard BPV underwent cutting balloon dilation followed by immediate conventional balloon pulmonary valvuloplasty.[33] This small case series revealed that the cutting balloon technique was safe and provided partial relief of resistant PS in children who failed standard BPV, avoiding the need for surgical intervention. Preliminary reports of cutting BPV in dogs with dysplastic PS have been published, suggesting fair to good outcomes can be achieved. The author has performed this technique in 8 dogs with fair to good results and no observable morbidity (**Fig. 4**). For sizing of cutting balloon dilation catheters, the author selects a cutting balloon diameter that is the same or 1 mm larger than the target site for dilation. Currently, cutting balloon and scoring balloon dilation catheters are available only up to 8 mm in diameter with a catheter lumen of 0.018 inch. A new device is in development that allows the operator to add scoring wires to any commercially available balloon dilation catheter, which may expand the utility of this technique to larger lesions. Early experience in the dog appears promising, but the device remains experimental.

When balloon dilation fails, surgical options should be considered. Stent implantation may provide an alternative therapeutic approach if surgery is not available or of too high a risk. Short-term results of 9 children with unsalvageable pulmonary valves and tetralogy of Fallot who underwent stenting across the pulmonary valve annulus

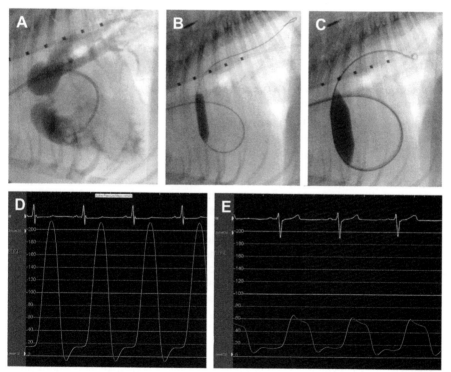

Fig. 4. Cutting and high-pressure BPV in a 6-month-old French bulldog with severe PS. The initial right ventriculogram (*A*) shows severe valve dysplasia with a segmental narrowing through the pulmonary valve. Cutting balloon dilation is performed over a 0.018-inch guidewire to score the lesion (*B*), followed by high-pressure balloon dilation (*C*). The pre-BPV right ventricular systolic pressure of 213 mm Hg (*D*) is reduced to 64 mm Hg after balloon (*E*), resulting in a 70% reduction that was confirmed by echocardiography the following day.

were promising.[34] More recently, a retrospective series of 52 children who underwent right ventricular stent implantation reported positive results for most patients, with 1 perioperative death related to pulmonary artery perforation.[35] Stent implantation at the pulmonary valve annulus has been reported in 2 dogs with an initial reduction in right ventricular pressure and transpulmonary gradient, as well as reduced clinical signs.[36] However, the improvement noted in each case was short-lived, with progressive in-stent stenosis due to muscular in-growth in one case and dynamic infundibular narrowing below the stent in the other.[36] A brief report described stent implantation for PS in an additional 3 dogs, with stent fracture occurring in 1 dog.[37] Sizing of the stent is not well defined in human reports, but most investigators report a stent diameter equal to or 1 to 2 mm larger than the diastolic pulmonary annular diameter.[38,39] Persistent muscular obstruction proximal to the stent also has been described,[40] and occurred in at least 2 of the reported canine cases.[36] Stent fracture is a concern when placing intracardiac stents related to the high forces exerted by the hypertrophied myocardium.[37,41] At this time, the author considers stent implantation for dogs with PS once they have failed high-pressure BPV, they have clinical signs or a high likelihood of an adverse outcome related to their PS, and when surgical therapies (patch graft, open surgical resection) are not available or desired by the client. When stent implantation is considered, the dog should be treated with an aggressive dose of beta-blockade to limit right ventricular contraction and lessen the risk of stent fracture. An atenolol dosage of 1.5 to 2.0 mg/kg by mouth every 12 hours is the target. **Figs. 5** and **6** demonstrate the procedure of balloon-expandable stent implantation in the pulmonary position for a dog with severe PS and right-sided heart failure that failed to improve after high-pressure BPV.

Does "Suicidal Right Ventricle" Occur in Dogs After Balloon Pulmonary Valvuloplasty and How Should It Be Treated?

The term suicidal right ventricle has been used in both human and veterinary literature to describe the phenomenon of a severe drop in cardiac output following BPV or during passage of wires through the right heart.[42,43] The acute reduction in resistance achieved with BPV unloads a right ventricle that is hypertrophied and acclimated to higher afterload. Severe muscular contraction of the right ventricular outflow tract can result, limiting right ventricular output and causing underfilling of the left heart with systemic arterial collapse. Although discussed in veterinary publications, the occurrence of true cardiovascular collapse immediately after BPV is quite rare. **Fig. 7** illustrates a case of severe PS (transpulmonary gradient by Doppler echocardiography of 256 mm Hg) in a 1.6 kg Pomeranian with a right-to-left shunting patent foramen ovale that became progressively hypoxemic after BPV with unmeasurable systemic blood pressure. Colloid and crystalloid infusion coupled with esmolol at 200 μg/kg per minute, diltiazem at 6 μg/kg per minute, and 3 boluses of dexmedetomidine at 0.5 μg/kg were required to restore systemic blood pressure. In general, therapy for systemic arterial collapse or marked hypoxemia after BPV should focus on expanding intravascular volume, limiting right ventricular contraction, and increasing systemic vascular resistance if a right-to-left shunting defect is present. Crystalloid or colloid boluses with esmolol administration as a 250 to 500 μg/kg intravenous bolus and continuous infusion at 75 to 150 μg/kg per minute works for most cases.

How Should Coronary Anatomy Be Evaluated in Dogs Before Balloon Pulmonary Valvuloplasty?

The association between PS and anomalous coronary artery anatomy was first reported by Buchanan and Patterson[44] in an English bulldog and further characterized

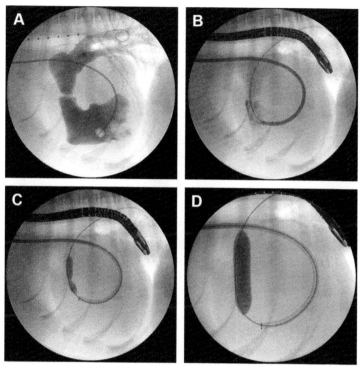

Fig. 5. Pulmonary valve stent implantation in a 6-month-old Staffordshire terrier. The dog had previously undergone BPV without improvement in the transpulmonary pressure gradient and was in right-sided congestive heart failure. The right ventriculogram (*A*) demonstrates right ventricular dilation with a dyskinetic and aneurysmal segment of the right ventricular freewall, as well as fused, thickened pulmonary valve leaflets. A long sheath is advanced to the right ventricular outflow tract, through which the balloon-expandable stent is advanced to the level of the pulmonary valve annulus (*B*). Inflation of the balloon on which the stent is mounted from the manufacturer is performed to plasty the stenotic valve to the side (*C*). In this case, a secondary overdilation was performed to bring the stent to the desired diameter (*D*).

in subsequent reports.[45,46] Additional reports in English bulldogs and boxer dogs have found alternative variants of the single coronary ostium.[47] Anomalous coronary arteries that encircle the pulmonary annulus are significant due to potential for damage during balloon valvuloplasty.[48] Diagnostic testing for anomalous coronary artery origin or course can include echocardiography, selective angiography, computed tomography (CT), and MRI. In the author's experience, transthoracic echocardiography can be suggestive of a single coronary ostium, but is not definitive. Transesophageal echocardiography is more capable of determining the origin and course of the coronary vessels than transthoracic imaging,[49] but is not as comprehensive as CT or MRI, which allows for volume-rendered 3-dimensional reformatting of the heart and a thorough evaluation of the origin and course of the major epicardial coronary arteries.[47,50] As the therapeutic options and the prognostic significance of correctly identifying a coronary artery anomaly in the setting of PS differ widely from a mistaken diagnosis, the author advises caution in making a definitive diagnosis by 2-dimensional echocardiography and still recommends angiography or cross-sectional imaging in most cases.

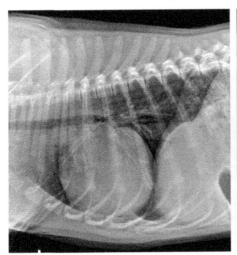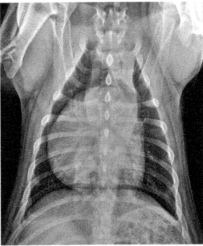

Fig. 6. Radiographs from the case in **Fig. 5** after pulmonary valve stent implantation. The dog's energy level improved poststenting and the transpulmonary valve pressure gradient reduced from 80 mm Hg to 50 mm Hg, in the setting of right ventricular dysfunction.

AORTIC AND SUBAORTIC STENOSIS

SAS is a common congenital defect of large-breed dogs; valvar aortic stenosis is more rarely encountered.[13,14,51] No therapy, medical,[52] transcatheter,[53] or surgical,[54] has shown a survival benefit for dogs with SAS, perhaps because the risk of sudden cardiac death is set before therapeutic intervention and cannot be altered with currently available strategies.

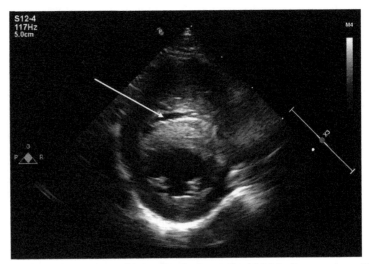

Fig. 7. Transverse echocardiographic image of a 5-month-old 1.6-kg Pomeranian with severe PS immediately following BPV. There is severe right ventricular hypertrophy with near obliteration of the right ventricular lumen (*arrow*). The transpulmonary valve pressure gradient in this dog reduced from 256 mm Hg preoperatively to 20 mm Hg after ballooning.

Which Patients Should Undergo Cutting and High-Pressure Balloon Dilation for Subaortic Stenosis?

The use of cutting and high-pressure balloon dilation for palliation of SAS has been described in dogs with fair short-term and mid-term results.[55–57] In an interim analysis of 28 dogs, a decrease in peak systolic pressure gradient was found from 143 mm Hg to 78 mm Hg at 1 day after ballooning, 84 mm Hg at 1 month, 89 mm Hg at 3 months, 92 mm Hg at 6 months, and 116 mm Hg at 12 months postprocedure.[57] Six dogs had died, including 3 dogs euthanized for progressive myocardial failure, 1 dog euthanized for syncope, and 2 dogs with sudden death.[57] The aortoseptal angle in dogs with SAS has been proposed to be predictive of balloon dilation efficacy, with angles narrower than 160° associated with less reduction in pressure gradient.[58] However, the correlations reported between aortoseptal angle, measured by angiography or echocardiography, and pressure gradient reduction were weak, suggesting this factor had limited predictive ability in determining outcome of intervention in the group studied. However, the idea warrants further evaluation in a larger population of dogs.

In the author's experience, having performed this procedure in 12 dogs, a reduction in gradient is achievable, and clients report improved exercise capacity, although a placebo effect cannot be excluded. The gradient typically reduces to the high moderate range (70–80 mm Hg) and obstruction persists. Long-term results remain unknown and no comparisons with medical therapy or the natural history of the disease have been made. A randomized prospective study is required to determine the benefit compared with medical therapy or no therapy.

It is the author's opinion that cases with a discrete subaortic ridge and minimal extension of fibrous tissue onto the anterior mitral valve leaflet are most amenable to successful intervention with cutting and high-pressure balloon valvuloplasty. The author's current preference is to select cases for intervention that have clinical signs (congestive heart failure, syncope, severe exercise intolerance) or echocardiographic changes that suggest clinical signs or a cardiac death are likely in the near term. The presence of clinical signs allows for an objective measure to gauge effectiveness of the intervention. The procedure is costly and involves risk, including arrhythmias, worsening of aortic insufficiency, and damage to the anterior mitral valve leaflet. In the absence of a study showing a survival benefit for cutting and high-pressure balloon intervention in SAS, a cautious approach to intervention may be the most prudent course.

Does Balloon Aortic Valvuloplasty Provide Any Relief of Valvar Aortic Stenosis in Dogs?

Although rare in the dog, valvar aortic stenosis is occasionally encountered. Commissural fusion and systolic doming are features of valvar aortic stenosis; a useful determinant of the level of obstruction by echo is noting where the flow turbulence initiates on color Doppler imaging. With SAS, flow acceleration and turbulence are noted below the aortic valve annulus and within the left ventricular outflow tract, whereas valvar aortic stenosis demonstrates flow acceleration and initiation of turbulence within the valve apparatus or at the leaflet tips.

Balloon dilation for SAS has been previously described.[56] The procedure for valvar aortic stenosis is similar, although cutting balloon dilation is not performed and the balloon is centered at the valve annulus rather than within the left ventricular outflow tract. A balloon-to-annulus ratio of approximately 1:1 is usually chosen to minimize stretch and potential damage to the aortic annulus, which may lead to worsening aortic insufficiency. The aortic annulus is best sized using the transthoracic or transesophageal echocardiographic long-axis image plane. Angiographic measurements of the true aortic annulus diameter during intervention can be challenging in dogs, as obtaining pure sagittal imaging by angiography is complicated by undefined fluoroscopic projections and cardiac remodeling. The author has used both low-pressure and high-pressure balloon dilation catheters for valvar aortic stenosis. Although no comparison is available, the author has observed better reductions in transvalvar gradients when using high-pressure balloons. **Fig. 8** demonstrates balloon aortic valvuloplasty in a 3-year-old Yorkshire terrier dog with a gradient of 200 mm Hg before balloon dilation, reduced to 70 mm Hg after high-pressure balloon aortic valvuloplasty.

PATENT DUCTUS ARTERIOSUS OCCLUSION

PDA is a common congenital heart defect in dogs, reported as the most common defect in some surveys.[12,59] It also occurs in cats, albeit with less frequency.[59] Without therapy, the prognosis is poor and closure of the ductus, either by surgical ligation or interventional occlusion, is therefore necessary.[60,61]

Transcatheter therapy for PDA was first reported in dogs in 1994.[62] In the initial decade of transcatheter PDA therapy, transarterial[3] or transvenous[63] coil delivery was the predominant method used for ductal closure. Thereafter, human implants

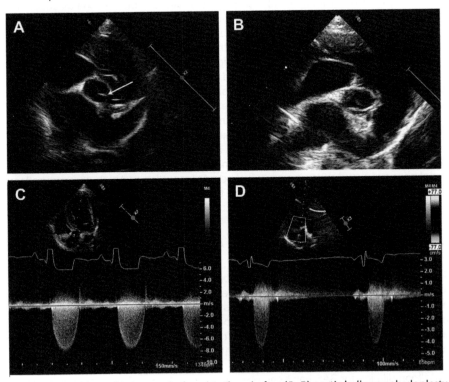

Fig. 8. Echocardiographic images before (A, C) and after (B, D) aortic balloon valvuloplasty in a Yorkshire terrier with valvar aortic stenosis. There is fusion along the commissure of the right and left adjacent aortic valve sinus (*arrow*), resulting in severe obstruction with a trans-aortic systolic pressure gradient of 200 mm Hg. Following high-pressure aortic balloon valvuloplasty, the commissure now opens and the gradient is reduced to 70 mm Hg for a 65% reduction.

of variable design[63–69] were reported for PDA occlusion in dogs, and in 2007 a device designed and optimized for canine anatomy was introduced.[70,71] The Canine Duct Occluder (CDO) is now the preferred transcatheter device for PDA occlusion in dogs due to an excellent safety and efficacy record and ease of deployment.[4] There remain a subset of small dogs, however, for which vascular access of sufficient size to deliver a CDO is not possible. A highly flexible nitinol device that can be delivered through smaller profile sheaths for small canine PDA has been evaluated with good results, but unfortunately is not available.[72]

What Are Transcatheter Options for Occlusion of Patent Ductus Arteriosus in Dogs Too Small for Canine Duct Occluder?

If the dog is too small for transarterial closure by CDO, surgical ligation by an experienced cardiothoracic surgeon should be considered. In general, CDO deployment will not be feasible if the femoral artery is too small to accept a 4-Fr or 5-Fr sheath; the smallest CDO devices can be delivered through a 4-Fr sheath, although 5-Fr access is often required. In the author's experience, it is feasible to achieve 4-Fr access in dogs that are at least 2.5 kg and 5-Fr access in dogs that are 3.5 kg and larger; however, this is not universally true and individual variation exists. Transvenous coil implantation allows for easier vascular access in small dogs, as the jugular or femoral vein are larger and more pliable than the femoral artery. Catheterization of the PDA from venous access requires placement of an end-hole catheter into the pulmonary trunk with a straight-tipped flexible guide wire advanced across the ductus to the descending aorta.[63,73] A detachable coil system is preferred to allow controlled release by exposing the coil in the descending aorta and withdrawing it into the ductal ampulla before release with a small segment of coil spanning the ductal ostium (**Fig. 9**).

In What Clinical Scenario Is Improving Ductal Flow Useful?

In some forms of congenital heart disease, preservation of the ductus arteriosus is useful to maintain sufficient pulmonary blood flow. Examples include pulmonary atresia with intact ventricular septum, tricuspid valve atresia, tetralogy of Fallot, and critical PS. In small animals, diagnosis of these severe defects rarely occurs in the neonatal period when ductal patency can be preserved. However, cases of cyanotic heart disease are occasionally seen in which the ductus arteriosus remains patent at the time of diagnosis. In such cases, stent implantation of the ductus may be considered as a less-invasive alternative to surgical creation of an aortopulmonary shunt. **Fig. 10** demonstrates the technique of ductal stenting in a dog with tetralogy of Fallot in which the diminutive ductus is crossed with a 0.014-inch coronary guidewire and then a 4 × 8-mm bare metal balloon-expandable stent is placed from the pulmonary trunk to the ductus, followed by coaxial placement of a second 4.5 × 13.0-mm stent throughout the ductal length. Under general anesthesia and with an inspired oxygen fraction of 100%, the dog's systemic arterial saturation rose from a Po_2 of 74 mm Hg to 289 mm Hg immediately after ductal stenting.

VASCULAR ACCESS AND CLOSURE

Every cardiac intervention short of hybrid surgical interventions requires peripheral vascular access to gain entry to the circulatory system. Venous access for interventional procedures is achieved percutaneously, or in some situations surgically, via the external jugular vein or the femoral vein in dogs and cats. Arterial access is almost universally achieved in animals by surgical cut-down to the femoral artery or common

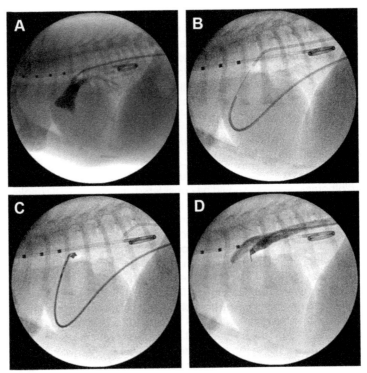

Fig. 9. Retrograde transvenous coil occlusion of PDA in a 13-week-old miniature Dachshund. The dog's femoral artery was deemed too small for an appropriate sheath to deliver a CDO, so transvenous, controlled coil delivery was performed. The initial angiogram (*A*) performed in the ductal ampulla shows a small left-to-right shunting ductus. A straight-tipped guidewire was used to cross the ductus from pulmonary trunk to aorta (*B*). The coil was partially extruded in the aorta and drawn back to engage the ductal ostium (*C*). Leaving a small portion of coil on the pulmonary side shows complete ductal occlusion on the post-coil angiogram (*D*).

carotid artery, This is in notable contrast to human medicine, in which arterial access is almost universally achieved through percutaneous femoral or radial arterial access.

How Best Should Vascular Access Be Achieved?

Effecting therapy through as minimal incision as possible is the hallmark of transcatheter therapies. As such, avoidance of surgical cut-down is desirable in animals both to reduce time of the procedure and for client perception. Furthermore, as current methods of surgical vascular access performed in animals often involve ligation of a major vessel at the procedure's end, a safe and effective percutaneous access route, with safe and effective closure of the arteriotomy/venotomy, could avoid this complication.

Although not widely reported in animals, ultrasound use during percutaneous vascular access provides several advantages. Ultrasound can be beneficial to confirm that the vessel intended for access is anatomically present and of sufficient caliber to accept the desired access sheath. Absence of an external jugular vein has been reported in both dogs and cats.[74,75] Ultrasound also is useful to guide vascular entry. Direct ultrasound guidance has been shown to improve percutaneous vascular access in human cardiac catheterization by reducing time to access, diminishing the number of attempts, and improving first-time success compared with palpation or

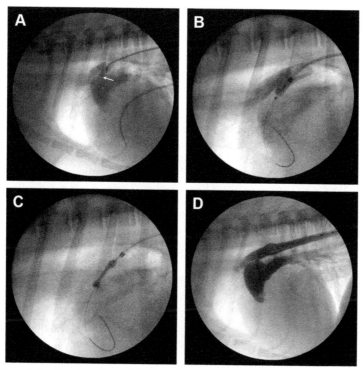

Fig. 10. Ductal stenting in a dog with clinical cyanosis and tetralogy of Fallot. An aortic injection into the ductal ampulla demonstrates a very small stream of contrast (*arrow*) through the PDA (*A*). After crossing the ductus with a 0.014-inch guidewire, the first balloon-expandable stent is positioned across the ductal ostium (*B*). As the first stent did not span the entire length of the ductus, a second stent is coaxially placed within the first and expanded (*C*). After stenting, a large stream of contrast can be seen through the ductus, resulting in improved pulmonary blood flow (*D*). A marked increased in systemic arterial saturation was noted on arterial blood gas analysis after stent implantation.

fluoroscopic guidance.[76] Ultrasound guidance for vascular access has not been well described or scientifically evaluated in animals, although experimental studies have demonstrated feasibility in dogs.[77] In the author's experience, ultrasound guidance is not typically required for external jugular venous access in dogs, although in dogs with very thick necks or extensive subcutaneous fat, it can be useful to confirm presence of the vessel and estimate depth from the skin. For femoral venous or arterial access in dogs, the author's experience has been that ultrasound guidance is helpful to establish the optimal path of needle access, to verify the desired vascular structure (artery or vein) is being selected, and to confirm entry to the vessel lumen. Subjectively, success during attempted access is improved compared with palpation-guided vascular access in the femoral triangle.

How Is Vascular Closure Best Achieved in Dogs and Cats Following Cardiac Intervention?

The author typically places a purse-string suture around the access tract after venous access, which is tightened as the sheath is removed. This suture can be removed in 12 to 24 hours and hemostasis is typically immediate, even with access up to 12-Fr. Arterial access in animals is complicated by an inability to easily limit patient movement and excitement after catheterization and therefore poses a high risk of hematoma formation at the access site if it is not closed directly. After arterial catheterization procedures in small animals, the femoral or carotid artery is ligated above and below the access site. In larger dogs, it can also be surgically repaired. Cats and dogs have sufficient collateral flow to allow ligation of either one or both common femoral arteries or a common carotid artery, although this limits ability to re-intervene and is, in the author's opinion, suboptimal for a procedure meant to be minimally invasive. The author has published successful use of a vascular closure device in a coagulopathic dog following percutaneous femoral arterial access,[78] which has become a common strategy in human medicine to minimize complications from manual compression and accelerate time to ambulation after percutaneous arterial access.[79] Several devices are available and result in effective hemostasis, allow for maintenance of arterial patency and preservation of the vessel, and avoid a surgical approach to the artery, thereby reducing pain/discomfort in recovery. Their use in veterinary medicine is untested, but may gain popularity in the future if safety and efficacy can be proven. An example of a suture-mediated vascular closure device after 12-Fr femoral venous access in a dog is shown in **Fig. 11**.

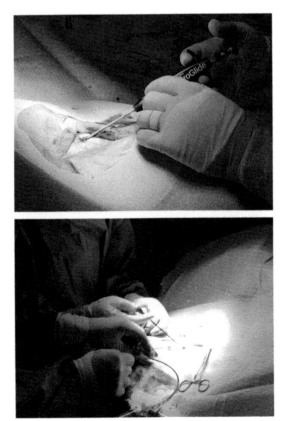

Fig. 11. Images during deployment of a suture-mediated vascular closure device after 12-Fr percutaneous access in the femoral vein of a dog. In the top image, the vascular closure device is advanced over a wire and the self-knotting suture is deployed through the venotomy. In the bottom image, following the intervention, the knot is tightened against the vessel wall as the sheath is removed and hemostasis is achieved.

SUMMARY

Interventional cardiology in veterinary medicine allows for the minimally invasive treatment of cardiac and vascular diseases in small animals. As the field matures, advances in device technology, patient selection, and procedural optimization should be pursued and scientifically evaluated. This article provides the author's perspective on common questions related to cardiac interventions, while highlighting areas in need of future study.

ACKNOWLEDGMENTS

The author gratefully acknowledges the assistance of John P. Cheatham, MD, during deployment of the ductal stents shown in **Fig. 10**, the assistance of John D. Carroll, MD, during deployment of the vascular closure device shown in **Fig. 11**, and the assistance of Marisa K. Ames, DVM, during the retrograde transvenous coil occlusion shown in **Fig. 9**.

REFERENCES

1. Scansen BA. Pulmonary valve stenosis. In: Weisse C, Berent A, editors. Veterinary image-guided interventions. Ames (IA): John Wiley & Sons, Ltd; 2015. p. 575–87.
2. Kleman ME. Aortic valve stenosis. In: Weisse C, Berent A, editors. Veterinary image-guided interventions. Ames (IA): John Wiley & Sons, Ltd; 2015. p. 588–94.
3. Gordon SG, Miller MW. Transarterial coil embolization for canine patent ductus arteriosus occlusion. Clin Tech Small Anim Pract 2005;20(3):196–202.
4. Gordon SG, Saunders AB, Achen SE, et al. Transarterial ductal occlusion using the Amplatz® canine duct occluder in 40 dogs. J Vet Cardiol 2010;12(2):85–92.
5. Stauthammer CD. Patent ductus arteriosus. In: Weisse C, Berent A, editors. Veterinary image-guided interventions. Ames (IA): John Wiley & Sons, Ltd; 2015. p. 564–74.
6. Saunders AB. Heartworm extraction. In: Weisse C, Berent A, editors. Veterinary image-guided interventions. Ames (IA): John Wiley & Sons, Ltd; 2015. p. 541–6.
7. Oyama MA, Sisson DD, Lehmkuhl LB. Practices and outcome of artificial cardiac pacing in 154 dogs. J Vet Intern Med 2001;15(3):229–39.
8. Hildebrandt N, Stertmann WA, Wehner M, et al. Dual chamber pacemaker implantation in dogs with atrioventricular block. J Vet Intern Med 2009;23(1):31–8.
9. Estrada AH. Cardiac pacing. In: Weisse C, Berent C, editors. Veterinary image-guided interventions. Ames (IA): John Wiley & Sons, Ltd; 2015. p. 518–30.
10. Musselman EE, Rouse GP, Parker AJ. Permanent pacemaker implantation with transvenous electrode placement in a dog with complete atrioventricular heart block, congestive heart failure and Stokes-Adams syndrome. J Small Anim Pract 1976;17(3):149–62.
11. Bright JM, Jennings J, Toal R, et al. Percutaneous balloon valvuloplasty for treatment of pulmonic stenosis in a dog. J Am Vet Med Assoc 1987;191(8):995–6.
12. Buchanan JW. Causes and prevalence of cardiovascular diseases. In: Kirk RW, Bonagura JD, editors. Current veterinary therapy XI: small animal practice. Philadelphia: WB Saunders Co; 1992. p. 647–54.
13. Oliveira P, Domenech O, Silva J, et al. Retrospective review of congenital heart disease in 976 dogs. J Vet Intern Med 2011;25(3):477–83.
14. Schrope DP. Prevalence of congenital heart disease in 76,301 mixed-breed dogs and 57,025 mixed-breed cats. J Vet Cardiol 2015;17(3):192–202.

15. Johnson MS, Martin M, Edwards D, et al. Pulmonic stenosis in dogs: balloon dilation improves clinical outcome. J Vet Intern Med 2004;18(5):656–62.
16. Francis AJ, Johnson MJ, Culshaw GC, et al. Outcome in 55 dogs with pulmonic stenosis that did not undergo balloon valvuloplasty or surgery. J Small Anim Pract 2011;52(6):282–8.
17. Ristic J, Marin C, Baines E, et al. Congenital pulmonic stenosis: a retrospective study of 24 cases seen between 1990–1999. J Vet Cardiol 2001;3(2):13–9.
18. Locatelli C, Spalla I, Domenech O, et al. Pulmonic stenosis in dogs: survival and risk factors in a retrospective cohort of patients. J Small Anim Pract 2013;54(9):445–52.
19. Schrope DP. Balloon valvuloplasty of valvular pulmonic stenosis in the dog. Clin Tech Small Anim Pract 2005;20(3):182–95.
20. Nomenclature ICoVGA. Nomina anatomica veterinaria. 6th edition. World Association of Veterinary Anatomists; 2017. Available at. http://www.wava-amav.org/wava-documents.html. Accessed June 1, 2018.
21. Bezuidenhout AJ. The heart and arteries. In: Evans HE, De Lahunta A, editors. Miller's anatomy of the dog. 4th edition. St Louis (MO): Elsevier Saunders; 2013. p. 428–504.
22. Keith A. The Hunterian lectures on malformations of the heart. Lancet 1909; 174(4484):359–63.
23. Lacour-Gayet F. Congenital heart surgery nomenclature and database project: right ventricular outflow tract obstruction-intact ventricular septum. Ann Thorac Surg 2000;69(4 Suppl):S83–96.
24. Detweiler DK. The heart. In: Hoskins HP, Lacroix JV, Mayer K, editors. Canine medicine. 2nd edition. Santa Barbara (CA): American Veterinary Publications, Inc; 1962. p. 275–358.
25. Patterson DF, Haskins ME, Schnarr WR. Hereditary dysplasia of the pulmonary valve in beagle dogs. Pathologic and genetic studies. Am J Cardiol 1981; 47(3):631–41.
26. Fathallah M, Krasuski RA. Pulmonic valve disease: review of pathology and current treatment options. Curr Cardiol Rep 2017;19(11):108.
27. Bussadori C, DeMadron E, Santilli RA, et al. Balloon valvuloplasty in 30 dogs with pulmonic stenosis: effect of valve morphology and annular size on initial and 1-year outcome. J Vet Intern Med 2001;15(6):553–8.
28. Moguillansky D, Schneider HE, Rome JJ, et al. Role of high-pressure balloon valvotomy for resistant pulmonary valve stenosis. Congenit Heart Dis 2010;5(2): 134–40.
29. Scansen BA. Interventional cardiology: what's new? Vet Clin North Am Small Anim Pract 2017;47(5):1021–40.
30. Belanger C, Gunther-Harrington CT, Nishimura S, et al. High-pressure balloon valvuloplasty for severe pulmonic stenosis: a prospective observational study in 25 dogs. J Vet Intern Med 2017;31(4):1243.
31. Yang SY, Qian CC, Hsia YF, et al. Transcatheter double-blade valvotomy for the treatment of valvar pulmonary stenosis. Pediatr Cardiol 1991;12(4):224–6.
32. Carlson KM, Neish SR, Justino H, et al. Use of cutting balloon for palliative treatment in tetralogy of Fallot. Catheter Cardiovasc Interv 2005;64(4):507–12.
33. Gavri S, Perles Z, Golender J, et al. Cutting balloon for the treatment of resistant pulmonic valve stenosis. Intervent Cardiol 2011;3(5):543–7.
34. Dohlen G, Chaturvedi RR, Benson LN, et al. Stenting of the right ventricular outflow tract in the symptomatic infant with tetralogy of Fallot. Heart 2009;95(2):142–7.
35. Stumper O, Ramchandani B, Noonan P, et al. Stenting of the right ventricular outflow tract. Heart 2013;99(21):1603–8.

36. Scansen BA, Kent AM, Cheatham SL, et al. Stenting of the right ventricular outflow tract in 2 dogs for palliation of dysplastic pulmonary valve stenosis and right-to-left intracardiac shunting defects. J Vet Cardiol 2014;16(3):205–14.
37. Swift S, Sosa I, Estrada A, et al. Stent angioplasty for treatment of balloon resistant canine valvular pulmonic stenosis. Paper presented at: ACVIM Forum. Indianapolis (IN), June 3–6, 2015.
38. Steadman CD, Clift PF, Thorne SA, et al. Treatment of dynamic subvalvar muscular obstruction in the native right ventricular outflow tract by percutaneous stenting in adults. Congenit Heart Dis 2009;4(6):494–8.
39. Castleberry CD, Gudausky TM, Berger S, et al. Stenting of the right ventricular outflow tract in the high-risk infant with cyanotic teratology of Fallot. Pediatr Cardiol 2013;35(3):423–30.
40. Barron DJ, Ramchandani B, Murala J, et al. Surgery following primary right ventricular outflow tract stenting for Fallot's tetralogy and variants: rehabilitation of small pulmonary arteries. Eur J Cardiothorac Surg 2013;44(4):656–62.
41. Nordmeyer J, Khambadkone S, Coats L, et al. Risk stratification, systematic classification, and anticipatory management strategies for stent fracture after percutaneous pulmonary valve implantation. Circulation 2007;115(11):1392–7.
42. Aprea F, Clark L, Whitley NT, et al. Presumed 'suicidal right ventricle' in a cocker spaniel dog undergoing pulmonary valve balloon dilation and its prevention in an analogous case. Vet Anaesth Analg 2014;41(4):438–9.
43. Singhal A, Kumar S, Kapoor A. Sudden iatrogenic suicidal right ventricle. Indian Heart J 2015;67(4):406–8.
44. Buchanan JW, Patterson DF. Selective angiography and angiocardiography in dogs with congenital cardiovascular disease. J Am Vet Radiol Soc 1965;6(1):21–39.
45. Buchanan JW. Pulmonic stenosis caused by single coronary artery in dogs: four cases (1965-1984). J Am Vet Med Assoc 1990;196(1):115–20.
46. Buchanan JW. Pathogenesis of single right coronary artery and pulmonic stenosis in English bulldogs. J Vet Intern Med 2001;15(2):101–4.
47. Scansen BA. Coronary artery anomalies in animals. Vet Sci 2017;4(2) [pii:E20].
48. Kittleson M, Thomas W, Loyer C, et al. Single coronary artery (type R2A). J Vet Intern Med 1992;6(4):250–1.
49. Navalon I, Pradelli D, Bussadori CM. Transesophageal echocardiography to diagnose anomalous right coronary artery type R2A in dogs. J Vet Cardiol 2015;17(4):262–70.
50. Laborda-Vidal P, Pedro B, Baker M, et al. Use of ECG-gated computed tomography, echocardiography and selective angiography in five dogs with pulmonic stenosis and one dog with pulmonic stenosis and aberrant coronary arteries. J Vet Cardiol 2016;18(4):418–26.
51. Lehmkuhl LB, Bonagura JD, Jones DE, et al. Comparison of catheterization and Doppler-derived pressure gradients in a canine model of subaortic stenosis. J Am Soc Echocardiogr 1995;8(5 Pt 1):611–20.
52. Eason BD, Fine DM, Leeder D, et al. Influence of beta blockers on survival in dogs with severe subaortic stenosis. J Vet Intern Med 2014;28(3):857–62.
53. Meurs KM, Lehmkuhl LB, Bonagura JD. Survival times in dogs with severe subvalvular aortic stenosis treated with balloon valvuloplasty or atenolol. J Am Vet Med Assoc 2005;227(3):420–4.
54. Orton EC, Herndon GD, Boon JA, et al. Influence of open surgical correction on intermediate-term outcome in dogs with subvalvular aortic stenosis: 44 cases (1991–1998). J Am Vet Med Assoc 2000;216(3):3.

55. Schmidt M, Estrada A, Maisenbacher Iii HW, et al. Combined cutting balloon and high pressure balloon angioplasty in dogs with severe subaortic stenosis is effective at mid-term follow-up. Catheter Cardiovasc Interv 2010;76(1):1.

56. Kleman ME, Estrada AH, Maisenbacher HW 3rd, et al. How to perform combined cutting balloon and high pressure balloon valvuloplasty for dogs with subaortic stenosis. J Vet Cardiol 2012;14(2):351–61.

57. Kleman ME, Estrada AH, Tschosik ML, et al. An update on combined cutting balloon and high pressure balloon valvuloplasty for dogs with severe subaortic stenosis. J Vet Intern Med 2013;27:632–3.

58. Shen L, Estrada AH, Cote E, et al. Aortoseptal angle and pressure gradient reduction following balloon valvuloplasty in dogs with severe subaortic stenosis. J Vet Cardiol 2017;19(2):144–52.

59. Scansen BA, Cober RE, Bonagura JD. Congenital heart disease. In: Bonagura JD, Twedt DC, editors. Kirk's current veterinary therapy XV. 15th edition. St Louis (MO): Saunders; 2014. p. 756–61.

60. Eyster GE, Eyster JT, Cords GB, et al. Patent ductus arteriosus in the dog: characteristics of occurrence and results of surgery in one hundred consecutive cases. J Am Vet Med Assoc 1976;168(5):435–8.

61. Saunders AB, Gordon SG, Boggess MM, et al. Long-term outcome in dogs with patent ductus arteriosus: 520 cases (1994-2009). J Vet Intern Med 2014;28(2):401–10.

62. Miller MW, Stepien RL, Meurs KM, et al. Echocardiographic assessment of patent ductus arteriosus (PDA) after occlusion. Proceedings of the 12th ACVIM Forum. San Francisco (CA), June 2–4, 1994.

63. Blossom JE, Bright JM, Griffiths LG. Transvenous occlusion of patent ductus arteriosus in 56 consecutive dogs. J Vet Cardiol 2010;12(2):75–84.

64. Grifka RG, Miller MW, Frischmeyer KJ, et al. Transcatheter occlusion of a patent ductus arteriosus in a Newfoundland puppy using the Gianturco-Grifka vascular occlusion device. J Vet Intern Med 1996;10(1):42–4.

65. Stokhof AA, Sreeram N, Wolvekamp WT. Transcatheter closure of patent ductus arteriosus using occluding spring coils. J Vet Intern Med 2000;14(4):452–5.

66. Sisson D. Use of a self-expanding occluding stent for nonsurgical closure of patent ductus arteriosus in dogs. J Am Vet Med Assoc 2003;223(7):999–1005.

67. Hogan DF, Green HW, Sanders RA. Transcatheter closure of patent ductus arteriosus in a dog with a peripheral vascular occlusion device. J Vet Cardiol 2006; 8(2):139–43.

68. Smith PJ, Martin MW. Transcatheter embolisation of patent ductus arteriosus using an Amplatzer vascular plug in six dogs. J Small Anim Pract 2007;48(2):80–6.

69. Achen SE, Miller MW, Gordon SG, et al. Transarterial ductal occlusion with the Amplatzer vascular plug in 31 dogs. J Vet Intern Med 2008;22(6):1348–52.

70. Nguyenba TP, Tobias AH. The Amplatz canine duct occluder: a novel device for patent ductus arteriosus occlusion. J Vet Cardiol 2007;9(2):109–17.

71. Nguyenba TP, Tobias AH. Minimally invasive per-catheter patent ductus arteriosus occlusion in dogs using a prototype duct occluder. J Vet Intern Med 2008; 22(1):129–34.

72. Olson JLC, Tobias AH, Stauthammer CD, et al. Minimally invasive per-catheter patent ductus arteriosus occlusion in small dogs (<3kg): preliminary results. J Vet Intern Med 2010;24(3):694.

73. Scansen BA. Cardiovascular interventional therapies. In: Ettinger SJ, Feldman EC, Cote E, editors. Textbook of veterinary internal medicine, vol. 1, 8th edition. St Louis (MO): Elsevier; 2017. p. 473–85.

74. Chapel EH, Scansen BA. Unilateral absence of an external jugular vein in two English bulldogs with pulmonary valve stenosis. J Vet Cardiol 2017;19(2):190–5.

75. Bertolini G, Zotti A. Imaging diagnosis: absence of the left external and both internal jugular veins in a cat. Vet Radiol Ultrasound 2006;47(5):468–9.

76. Seto AH, Abu-Fadel MS, Sparling JM, et al. Real-time ultrasound guidance facilitates femoral arterial access and reduces vascular complications: FAUST (Femoral Arterial Access with Ultrasound Trial). JACC Cardiovasc Interv 2010; 3(7):751–8.

77. Chamberlin SC, Sullivan LA, Morley PS, et al. Evaluation of ultrasound-guided vascular access in dogs. J Vet Emerg Crit Care (San Antonio) 2013;23(5): 498–503.

78. Scansen BA, Hokanson CM, Friedenberg SG, et al. Use of a vascular closure device during percutaneous arterial access in a dog with impaired hemostasis. J Vet Emerg Crit Care (San Antonio) 2017;27(4):465–71.

79. Schwartz BG, Burstein S, Economides C, et al. Review of vascular closure devices. J Invasive Cardiol 2010;22(12):599–607.

Interventional Radiology Management of Vascular Obstruction

Marilyn Dunn, DVM, MVSc[a], Brian A. Scansen, DVM, MS[b],*

KEYWORDS

• Canine • Feline • Intervention • Stent • Angioplasty • Coagulation • Thrombosis

KEY POINTS

• Vascular obstructions may develop secondary to intraluminal obstruction or extraluminal compression, with thrombosis a common sequela.

• Interventional options for vascular obstruction include catheter-directed thrombolysis, angioplasty, and vascular stenting. Concurrent medical management of thrombosis is required, involving antiplatelet and anticoagulant therapy.

• Acute presentation of vascular obstruction requires urgent intervention both to improve vascular flow and to prevent thrombus maturation that may limit response to therapy.

• Dogs and cats with more chronic, insidious signs of vascular obstruction may have a good outcome with medical therapy alone.

INTRODUCTION

Vascular obstructions may result from intraluminal obstruction (thrombus, neoplasia, foreign body) or from extraluminal compression (neoplasia, malformation, granuloma) resulting in altered blow flow downstream and congestion upstream of the obstruction. Regardless of underlying cause, thrombosis often occurs secondary to the altered flow dynamics present in an obstruction.

In veterinary medicine, thrombosis is recognized as a common complication of many acquired diseases, including cardiac, endocrine, immunologic, inflammatory, and neoplastic disorders (**Table 1**).[1] Due to challenges in confirming the diagnosis

Disclosure Statement: Dr M. Dunn has no conflicts to disclose. Dr B.A. Scansen has received speaking fees, travel reimbursement, or product at no cost for development/preclinical evaluation from the following companies relevant to this publication: Infiniti Medical, LLC; Avalon Medical, Inc; and Dextronix, Inc.
 a Interventional Radiology and Endoscopy, CHUV- Faculty of Veterinary Medicine, University of Montreal, 3200 Sicotte, St. Hyacinthe, Quebec J2S 7C6, Canada; b Cardiology and Cardiac Surgery, Department of Clinical Sciences, Colorado State University, Campus Delivery 1678, Fort Collins, CO 80523, USA
* Corresponding author.
E-mail address: Brian.Scansen@colostate.edu

Vet Clin Small Anim 48 (2018) 819–841
https://doi.org/10.1016/j.cvsm.2018.05.004
0195-5616/18/© 2018 Elsevier Inc. All rights reserved.

Table 1		
Common conditions associated with venous and arterial thrombosis in dogs and cats		
	Dog	Cat
Arterial	Protein-losing nephropathy Hyperadrenocorticism Neoplasia Immune-mediated disease (eg, hemolytic anemia) Glucocorticoid therapy	Left-sided cardiovascular disease Pulmonary neoplasia
Venous	Adrenal neoplasia Liver disease (inflammatory, neoplastic, other) Immune-mediated disease (hemolytic anemia, etc)	Adrenal neoplasia Liver disease (inflammatory, neoplastic, other)
Mixed (including pulmonary thromboembolism)	Sepsis Pancreatitis Immune-mediated disease (eg, hemolytic anemia)	Sepsis Pancreatitis

of vascular obstruction and thrombosis in veterinary medicine, it is likely that many patients go undiagnosed, making the true prevalence of these conditions difficult to estimate. Even when the presence of an obstruction or thrombus is confirmed, limited therapeutic options and confusion regarding medical management leads to uncertainty in treatment plans. A multimodal approach involving a combination of interventional radiology, antiplatelet therapy, anticoagulant therapy, and thrombolytics likely holds the greatest promise for management of vascular obstructions in small animal patients.

This article describes interventional options for vascular obstructions including arterial, central venous, and portal obstructions. No large-scale prospective studies have evaluated these techniques or therapeutic strategies in animals; therefore, this article represents the authors' opinion and clinical experience in managing these conditions.

GENERAL CONSIDERATION FOR VASCULAR OBSTRUCTIONS

Normal hemostasis is maintained through a delicate balance between endogenous anticoagulants and procoagulants. The net effect is preservation of blood flow in the systemic vasculature with localized coagulation at sites of vessel injury. Changes in this balance can tip to either excessive bleeding or thrombus formation, depending on underlying disease state. The primary disorder influences the site of thrombus formation (arterial or venous) as well as the composition of the occluding thrombus. The relative proportions of platelets and fibrin in the thrombus depend on the shear forces within the injured vessel. Arterial thrombi form under high shear forces and therefore tend to contain a large number of platelets held together by fibrin strands. Venous thrombi form under low shear forces and consist primarily of fibrin and red blood cells. Mixed thrombi are an intermediate form and occur in the pulmonary vasculature. Some of these long-held beliefs are now being challenged and the role of platelets in venous thrombosis may have been underestimated.[2] Strategies to inhibit arterial thrombogenesis typically include the use of antiplatelet drugs, whereas anticoagulants are the mainstay of venous thromboprophylaxis.

An important consideration in the decision-making process in a thrombotic patient is the site of the thrombus. An arterial thrombus is often considered an emergency and time to intervention is critical unless collateral circulation is present (or has developed). Venous thrombosis may present less acutely or be found incidentally, making the need for immediate intervention more difficult to ascertain. For instance, in a patient with a partially obstructive vena caval thrombus and minimal or no venous congestion, medical management of the underlying prothrombotic state may allow the patient's fibrinolytic system to slowly eliminate the obstruction, although subsequent migration or embolism of the thrombus must be considered.[3,4]

AORTIC OBSTRUCTION

Aortic obstruction in animals is typically intraluminal, as the high arterial pressure limits extraluminal compression. In small animals, aortic obstructions occur secondary to a cardiogenic embolus, dissection of the arterial wall, intravascular neoplasia, or in situ thrombosis. The cat is almost exclusively affected by cardiogenic emboli in the setting of myocardial disease, left atrial enlargement, and blood stasis in the left auricular appendage.[5,6] Dogs appear to develop aortic thrombosis in situ secondary to a prothrombotic state such as protein-losing nephropathy, recent steroid administration, endocrinopathy, infective endocarditis, or neoplasia.[7–11] The Shetland sheepdog has been identified as a breed at increased risk for aortic thrombosis[11]; anecdotally, greyhound dogs also appear to be at increased for idiopathic aortic thrombosis. In some canine cases for which an underlying systemic disease resulting in a prothrombotic state cannot be identified, the aortic lesion, including site and extent of thrombus, resembles Leriche syndrome in humans, also known as aortoiliac occlusive disease.[12] Aortoiliac occlusive disease is associated with severe arteriosclerotic narrowing or occlusion of the infrarenal aorta and iliac arteries, which is also the most common site of aortic thrombosis in the dog in the authors' experience. Additionally, postmortem evaluation of dogs affected with aortic thrombosis in the authors' practice have demonstrated marked intimal degeneration and thickening compatible with severe arteriosclerotic changes to the aortic wall. Whether these changes initiated the thrombus or occurred secondary to the presence of thrombus is unclear. Although rare, aortic obstruction may also develop in both the dog and cat secondary to an aortic dissection with expansion and occasional thrombosis of the false lumen created by the dissection (**Fig. 1**).[13] Intra-aortic neoplasia may also lead to aortic obstruction, which has been reported in dogs with both angiosarcoma and chrondrosarcoma.[14,15]

Many dogs present with signs of claudication (**Fig. 2**) and limited exercise capacity; although occasionally the thrombus is detected incidentally. In one case series, 20 of 26 dogs were ambulatory at the time of diagnosis and most were managed effectively with oral anticoagulant therapy.[7] Conversely, other case series describe marked differences in survival between those with a chronic history (median survival of 293 days after treatment) compared with those with an acute presentation (9 days).[9] A review article noted that most studies demonstrate a 50% to 60% rate of survival from presentation to discharge for dogs with aortic thrombosis.[10] In the cat, the severity of the underlying heart disease, acuity of clinical signs, and high rate of ischemia-reperfusion injury result in a guarded to poor prognosis. Historically, only a third of cats survive the initial arterial thromboembolic episode; however, survival statistics improve when cats euthanized without therapy are excluded or when only cases from recent years are analyzed.[6,16,17] Survival is better if only one limb is involved and/or if some motor function is preserved at presentation.[6]

The optimal therapy for aortic obstruction in dogs and cats is ill-defined. Currently, cats are treated with medical therapy and interventional strategies are not pursued.[5] Rheolytic thrombectomy has been reported to have a high success rate for

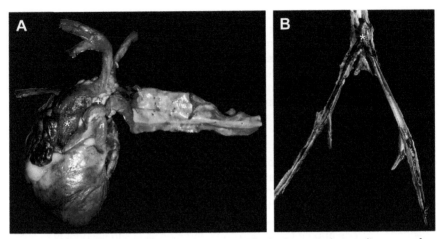

Fig. 1. Postmortem images of aortic obstruction. (*A*) The heart and ascending aorta from a cat with systemic hypertension that developed aortic dissection with thrombosis (*asterisk*) of the false lumen, which resulted in compression and partial obstruction of the true aortic lumen (*plus*). (*B*) The distal aorta, iliac, and femoral arteries from a dog with aortoiliac thrombosis. The thrombus (*asterisk*) was present in the terminal aorta and extended down both rear limbs.

establishing revascularization in a pilot study of 5 of 6 cats, but survival to discharge (50%) was comparable to medical therapy alone and therefore is not advised.[18] The authors advise medical therapy, a combination antiplatelet and anticoagulant medications with physical therapy and supportive care, in dogs diagnosed with aortic thrombosis and a chronic history that remain ambulatory. Antiplatelet doses of clopidogrel at 2 mg/kg by mouth every 24 hours coupled with an oral anticoagulant is the typical approach. Considerations for anticoagulation include unfractionated heparin, low molecular weight heparin (LMWH), warfarin, and new oral anticoagulants such as rivaroxaban and apixaban. Use of a heparin continuous rate infusion has been advocated for short-term management of thrombotic disease at a dosage of 25 to 50 U/kg per hour, typically targeting a 1.5 to 2.0 times increase in the activated partial thromboplastic

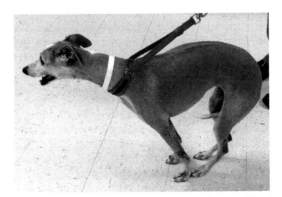

Fig. 2. A dog with aortic thrombosis after a walk. Note the hunched back and reluctance to bear weight in the rear limbs.

time (aPTT) from baseline.[4] Activated clotting time is not recommended to monitor chronic heparin therapy, but can be useful intraoperatively during catheter-based procedures, although the ideal target in dogs or cats is unknown (times of 250–400 seconds are often used during arterial interventions in humans). Hemorrhage is the major complication of unfractionated heparin, given its complex pharmacodynamics. Unfortunately, monitoring of aPTT and anti-Xa activity has not proven sufficiently accurate to predict efficacy and bleeding risk during heparin therapy.[19] LMWHs have greater bioavailability and a longer half-life than unfractionated heparin when given subcutaneously, because of lesser binding to plasma proteins as well as endothelial cells and macrophages.[20] Dalteparin sodium has been used in animals (100–150 U/kg subcutaneously [SC] every 8–24 hours), but some animals may require more frequent dosing.[21–23] Enoxaparin has been advised at 1 mg/kg SC every 12 hours. Predicted feline doses to maintain anti-Xa activity within (human) therapeutic range have been suggested as 150 IU/kg SC every 4 hours for dalteparin, and 1.5 mg/kg SC every 6 hours for enoxaparin.[24] However, such doses may not be necessary for antithrombotic activity, as enoxaparin (1 mg/kg SC every 12 hours) had significant antithrombotic effect for at least 12 hours with no correlation between plasma anti-Xa activity and thrombus formation in a feline venous thrombosis model.[25] Warfarin therapy is complicated by variable absorption and frequent monitoring, although the drug itself is of low cost. Typical dosing is 0.1 to 0.2 mg/kg by mouth every 24 hours, with adjustments made on a weekly basis to target international normalized ratio of 2 to 3.[7] New oral anticoagulants are available that do not require injection, have a relatively predictable pharmacodynamic profile, and have shown superiority to chronic warfarin therapy in limiting cardiogenic thromboembolic disease in people.[26–28] These agents include the direct thrombin inhibitor dabigatran and the factor Xa inhibitors rivaroxaban and apixaban. Studies are limited in animals, but rivaroxaban has been used in dogs at doses of roughly 0.5 to 1 mg/kg by mouth every 24 hours, whereas experimental studies and other investigators suggest a dosage of 2 mg/kg by mouth every 12 hours.[4,29–31] Studies in healthy cats suggest rivaroxaban is tolerated at dosages of 1.25 mg by mouth every 12 hours and 2.5 mg by mouth every 24 hours; twice-daily dosing of 1.25 mg or 2.5 mg per cat may be preferable to once-daily dosing based on anti-factor Xa activity.[32] Studies of apixaban in healthy cats showed that oral and intravenous dosing at 0.2 mg/kg reduced factor Xa activity, but chronic oral dosing studies are not available.[33] One of the authors (BAS) has used apixaban in dogs at doses up to 0.5 mg/kg by mouth every 8 to 12 hours without severe side effects, although optimal dosing for thrombotic disease is unknown.

Dogs that have a more acute presentation or signs of distal limb ischemia likely require intervention to improve what are poor survival statistics. However, the optimal interventional therapy for aortic thrombosis in dogs is not clear. Rheolytic thrombectomy and vascular stenting at the aortic trifurcation have been described in dogs with aortic thrombosis.[4] However, restoration of flow is paramount to achieving a sustainable result, as the best antithrombotic is the elimination of stasis and restoration of blood flow. In some dogs with aortic thrombosis, the internal iliac system as well as the external iliac, femoral, and distal branch arteries are affected (see **Fig. 1**). If access to a patent lumen beyond the distal obstruction cannot be achieved, either through distal vascular access or guidewire navigation through the obstruction, stenting of the proximal inflow portion may not be effective (**Fig. 3**). Additionally, in acute thrombosis, the presence of soft thrombus may simply squish through the interces of a stent and result in continued luminal obstruction (**Fig. 4**). Cross-sectional imaging, either computed tomography angiography or magnetic resonance angiography, can be very useful to determine the extent of thrombosis as well as the presence of distal

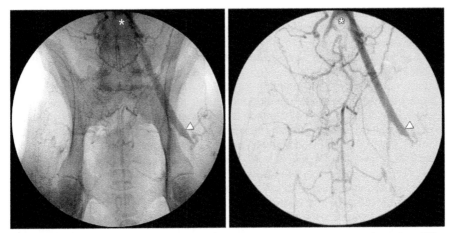

Fig. 3. Distal aortic angiogram from a dog with aortoiliac thrombosis. There is a filling defect at the aortic trifurcation (*asterisk*) with complete occlusion of the right external iliac artery and occlusion of the left femoral artery just distal to the origin of the left deep femoral artery (*arrowhead*). Without filling of the femoral vessels below these sites of obstruction, angioplasty or vascular stenting above these sites (eg, at the aortoiliac junction) is unlikely to provide relief of acute hindlimb ischemia.

arterial patency (**Fig. 5**). Currently, the authors' approach to acute limb ischemia in the dog is to evaluate for the presence of underlying disease, determine the extent of obstruction in the distal vascular bed, and attempt to establish revascularization. Surgical thrombectomy, rheolytic thrombectomy, or catheter (Fogarty) thrombectomy may all be considered, depending on the available expertise. In addition, interventional options such as catheter-directed thrombolysis, angioplasty, or stent implantation may be considered. For acute thrombosis, infusion of recombinant tissue plasminogen activator (tPA) throughout the site of thrombosis for 24 to 48 hours might be useful to lyse all soft thrombus while systemic heparin is provided to reduce future thrombus formation. The use of infusion catheters (**Fig. 6**), termed catheter-directed thrombolysis, can help to deliver the lytic agent diffusely throughout the thrombus, which may be preferable to infusing the entire dose at the proximal or distal aspect of the thrombus where it may only bind to the exposed end. The thrombolytic tPA is given as a continuous infusion at 0.5 to 1.0 mg/h for 24 to 48 hours through an infusion catheter, which bathes the thrombus in the lytic agent throughout its full extent while reducing systemic risk of bleeding, as lower doses of tPA are given than would be chosen for systemic dosing. Follow-up angiography to determine extent of remaining disease after lysis can then dictate optimal sites for angioplasty or stenting. To the authors' knowledge, this approach has not been rigorously evaluated in small animal patients and is complicated by the difficulties in managing the dog or cat with indwelling arterial infusion catheters for a prolonged period of time. Angioplasty may be considered if the thrombus is adherent to vessel wall and dislodgement and distal embolization are considered low risk. A well-organized thrombus or site of extraluminal compression may be treated by implantation of a bare metal or covered stent. Covered stents are available on the human market with a heparin-impregnated coating to limit thrombotic occlusion, but their use has not been reported in animals. A covered stent, or stent graft, may be used to limit the risk of thrombus extruding through the interces of the stent if the maturity of the lesion is unknown. Optimal staging of these procedures and preferred case selection for each remains uncertain.

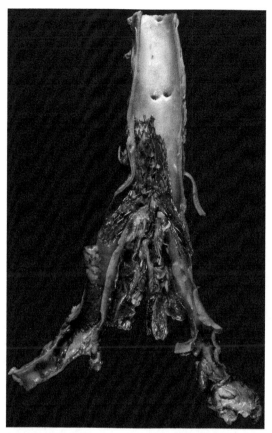

Fig. 4. Postmortem photograph of the terminal aorta from the dog in **Fig. 3**. Stenting in an area of acute, soft thrombus results in extrusion of the thrombus through the interces of the stent with continued obstruction. The distal right iliac and left femoral arteries remain occluded such that improvement of the inflow portion to the iliofemoral system will not result in resolution of distal limb ischemia unless distal outflow can be achieved.

CENTRAL VENOUS OBSTRUCTION

Obstruction of small or peripheral veins likely occurs in dogs with regularity secondary to trauma, phlebitis, or indwelling catheters. However, clinical signs related to venous obstruction seldom develop, due to extensive collateral pathways for venous return,[34,35] until central venous obstruction occurs (**Fig. 7**). Central venous obstruction implies stenosis or occlusion of the major veins (left and right subclavian veins, left and right brachiocephalic veins, left and right common iliac veins, and the cranial and caudal vena cava). Obstruction of these veins may occur secondary to extraluminal compression,[34–37] congenital malformations,[34,38–40] intravascular foreign bodies (indwelling catheters, pacemaker leads),[41–43] large-volume abdominal effusion,[44] trauma,[45,46] phlebitis,[47] thrombosis,[48–50] or neoplasia.[34,51,52]

The interventional management of central venous obstruction depends on the etiology, chronicity, location, underlying disease prognosis, and client desire. Congenital malformations that result in impaired venous return typically affect the caudal vena cava and lead to ascites. A divided right atrium, also known as cor triatriatum dexter

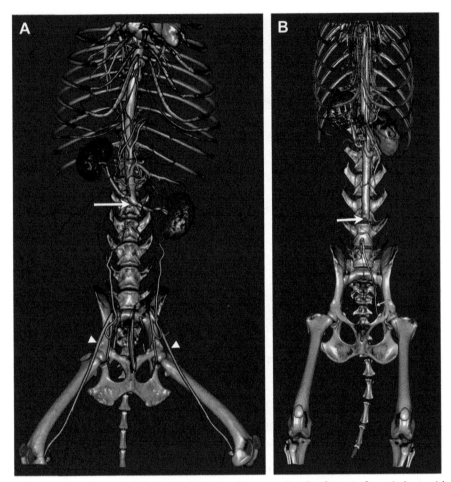

Fig. 5. Computed tomography angiographic volume-rendered reformats from 2 dogs with aortoiliac thrombosis. In the case (*A*), the contrast column in the aorta ends just beyond the renal arteries (*arrow*) yet flow is apparent through superficial epigastric collateral arteries perfusing the femoral arteries (*arrowheads*) and distal pelvic limbs. In contrast, case (*B*) shows a dog with thrombosis at the caudal aorta (*arrow*) without any apparent contrast filling of the external iliac arteries or femoral arteries, with only patency of the left internal iliac artery (*small arrow*) demonstrated.

(CTD), and Budd-Chiari–like membranes obstructing hepatic venous outflow are the more commonly encountered congenital causes. Balloon dilation of CTD was reported in 2 dogs in 1999,[53,54] with additional successful cases reported thereafter, but balloon dilation was unsuccessful in a cat with a Budd-Chiari–like lesion.[55] Balloon membranostomy is often performed first for these defects, although in the authors' experience and in anecdotal reports[56] it does not always provide a permanent resolution, and uncontrolled fracture of the membrane can be dangerous.[55] The use of cutting balloon dilation for CTD was reported in 2012 in 2 dogs and theorized to create a more controlled initial cut in the membrane, to be extended by conventional balloon dilation.[56] The authors now use cutting balloon followed by high-pressure balloon dilation in most membranostomy cases to create a controlled and complete tear in the

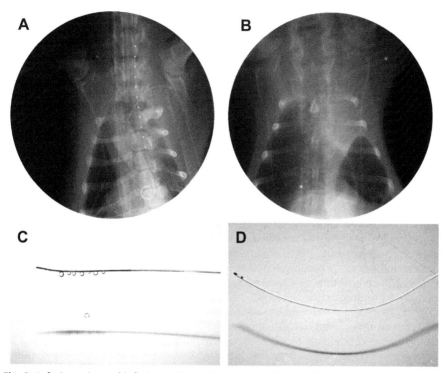

Fig. 6. Infusion wire and infusion catheter for catheter-directed thrombolysis. Infusion wires are small-diameter (0.035-inch), single-lumen, closed-end wires with multiple side holes and a Luer lock adapter at the end. (*A*) An infusion wire positioned across the left brachiocephalic vein of a dog. (*C*) Close-up picture of the distal end of an infusion wire with saline being infused. Infusion catheters are catheters of variable size that can be passed over a guidewire with multiple side holes, but with a valve at the catheter tip to prevent infusion through the end hole. (*B*) An infusion catheter positioned across the left brachiocephalic vein of a dog. (*D*) A close-up picture of the distal end of an infusion catheter with saline being infused. In both (*A*) and (*C*), the radiopaque markers illustrate the length of the infusion area.

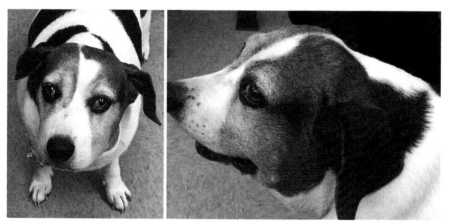

Fig. 7. A dog with thrombosis of the cranial vena cava, resulting in facial swelling, prolapse of the nictitating membranes, and ventral cervical edema.

membrane (**Fig. 8**). The cutting balloon dilation catheter is sized at a 4 to 8-mm diameter by 2-cm length in most dogs or at least 1 mm larger than an echocardiographic measure of the membrane ostium, if known. A high-pressure balloon dilation catheter then follows, which is typically sized 1:1 to the maximal diameter of the caudal vena cava as measured on predilation venography. It may not be necessary to use high-pressure balloon dilation after cutting balloon dilation; conventional balloon dilation catheters were used in the original report.[56] However, the membrane of CTD on postmortem can be muscular or fibromuscular and it is the authors' opinion that high-pressure dilation provides a more effective tear. In some cases, cutting and high-pressure balloon dilation do not sufficiently dilate the membrane or provide a lasting resolution to caudal venous obstruction. In such cases, intravascular stent implantation has been described[57–59] and is the authors' preferred treatment strategy.

Sclerosis and thrombosis of the central veins is commonly associated with dialysis grafts and central venous catheterization in humans.[60] The spectrum of etiologies causing venous thrombosis is not as well-defined in animals, although in the authors' experience can occur with indwelling central venous catheters, chronic vascular implants, such as sampling ports or pacemaker leads, prior surgery involving the vein or nearby structures, or extension of thrombus into the vein from local neoplastic disease, as with adrenal tumors. These etiologies are more likely to result in thrombosis if a concurrent prothrombotic systemic disease is present, such as protein-losing nephropathy or hyperadrenocorticism. Management of central venous thrombosis leading to limb swelling, head edema, or cavitary effusion should be prompt and initiated as soon as the condition is recognized; delays in intervention allow the thrombus to organize and mature, which may limit potential response to therapy. If the duration of thrombus is known to be acute (less than a week and optimally <48 hours), lytic therapies may be considered using tPA. Delivery of tPA may be either systemic, given nonselectively into a peripheral vein, or local, given directly at the site of thrombus. No studies have evaluated either approach in small animals, but the authors' preference is to deliver tPA locally to avoid dilutional effects and reduce the total dose required. Systemic doses of 0.5 to 1.0 mg/kg tPA infused over 30 to 60 minutes have been described in dogs and cats; a graduated bolus/infusion approach has also been proposed (**Table 2**). With catheter-directed therapy, 2 to 8 mg total per animal of tPA is infused as close to the site of thrombus as possible. Alternatively, prolonged instillation through an infusion catheter may be considered, with tPA given as a continuous infusion at 0.5 to 1.0 mg/h for 24 to 48 hours.[61] This strategy appears effective in deep venous thrombosis of humans.[61] Newer devices are available that both infuse thrombolytic and also mechanically agitate the thrombus with the ability to aspirate debris during the procedure. To the authors' knowledge, these devices have not been evaluated in small animal patients.

In cases that fail thrombolysis, venoplasty or venous stenting may be considered. Balloon venoplasty involves dilating the venous lumen. It is often considered following thrombolysis, as the lytic agent should have allowed dissolution of acute thrombus and what remains is likely adherent to the vessel wall, of chronic duration, and may continue to obstruct or serve as a nidus for recurrent thrombosis. Balloon venoplasty for central venous obstruction in a dog is shown in **Fig. 9**. When balloon venoplasty fails, a resistant stricture is present, or continued extraluminal compression is likely, venous stent implantation may be considered. Stent implantation allows for continued radial force to be exerted at the site of obstruction and may help to maintain venous patency. Venous stenting for vascular obstructions in small animals is in its infancy, but an example of restored patency after stent implantation and secondary dilation is shown in **Fig. 10**. Antithrombotic therapy (unfractionated heparin, LMWH, or factor

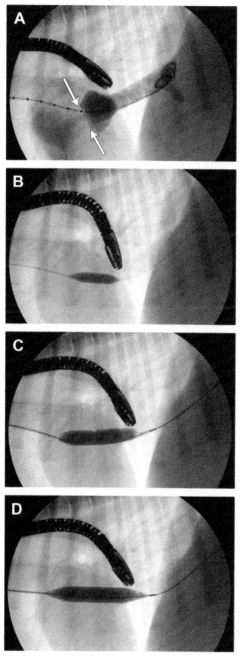

Fig. 8. Fluoroscopic images during cutting and high-pressure balloon dilation of CTD in a dog with ascites. The initial angiogram (A) demonstrates a perforate membrane (between *arrows*) in the caudal right atrium, which is limiting caudal venous return. Scoring of the membrane is performed with a cutting balloon dilation catheter (B), followed by high-pressure balloon dilation that initially demonstrates a stenotic waist (C) which resolves on full inflation (D). A transesophageal echocardiography probe is present in all images. The dog's ascites resolved after the procedure.

Table 2
Anticoagulant, antiplatelet, and thrombolytic (fibrinolytic) drugs commonly used in small animal patients and the recommended doses and frequency of administration

Drug	Dog	Cat
Anticoagulants		
Unfractionated heparin	150–300 units/kg SC q8 h CRI 25–50 units/kg/h[a] Adjust to achieve 1.5–2.0 times baseline PTT values	250–300 units/kg SC q8 h CRI 25–50 units/kg/h[a] Adjust to achieve 1.5–2.0 times baseline PTT values
Low molecular weight heparin		
Dalteparin	150 units/kg SC q8–24 h[a]	150 units/kg SC q6–12 h[a]
Enoxaparin	0.8 mg/kg SC q6 h[a]	1.5 mg/kg SC q6 h[a]
Factor Xa inhibitors		
Rivaroxaban	1–2 mg/kg PO q12–24 h[a]	1.25, 2.5, and 5.0 mg/cat q12h for 3 d, then 2.5 mg q24h for 7 d, then 1.25 mg q24h for 28 d[a]
Apixaban	0.25–0.5 mg/kg PO q8–12 h[a]	0.625–1.25 mg/cat q12 h[a]
Warfarin	0.2 mg/kg PO q24 h Adjust to INR of 2–3	0.5 mg/cat PO q24 h Adjust to achieve 1.5–2.0 times baseline PT values
Antiplatelets		
Acetylsalicylic acid	0.5 mg/kg PO q12 h	5 mg/cat PO q72 h
Clopidogrel	1–2 mg/kg PO q24 h	18.75 mg/cat PO q24 h
Thrombolytics		
IV dose can be given directly at the site of the thrombus		
Tissue plasminogen activator	0.5 mg/kg IV over 30–60 min 0.2 mg/kg IV bolus, then 0.7 mg/kg IV over 30 min, then 0.5 mg/kg IV over 1 h (1.4 mg/kg Total Dose) Can be repeated up to 3 times within 24 h[b]	0.5 mg/kg IV over 30–60 min 0.75 mg IV bolus, then 2.5 mg IV over 30 min, then 1.75 mg IV over 1 h (5 mg Total Dose) Can be repeated up to 3 times within 24 h
Streptokinase	90,000 units IV over 30 min followed by CRI of 45,000 units/h IV over 6–12 h	90,000 units IV over 30 min followed by CRI of 45, 000 units/h IV over 6–12 h

Abbreviations: CRI, constant rate infusion; INR, international normalized ratio; IV, intravenous; PO, by mouth; PT, prothrombin time; PTT, partial thromboplastin; q, every; SC, subcutaneous.
[a] Please note that these doses have been taken from abstracts and personal data and are largely unpublished.
[b] The authors have never used more than 9 mg per dog for systemic dosing.

Xa inhibitor) with or without antiplatelet therapy (clopidogrel, aspirin) is usually required concurrent with thrombolytic or interventional therapy.

Tumors within or adjacent to the heart can result in obstruction to venous return.[52] Intracardiac or intravascular stent implantation can palliate clinical signs in affected dogs and may prolong survival.[37,62,63] Successful resolution of pleural effusion after venous stenting secondary to heart base tumors and obstruction of the cranial vena cava was recently reported in 2 dogs.[37] Transatrial stent implantation for right atrial tumors that result in caudal or cranial vena caval obstruction (**Fig. 11**)

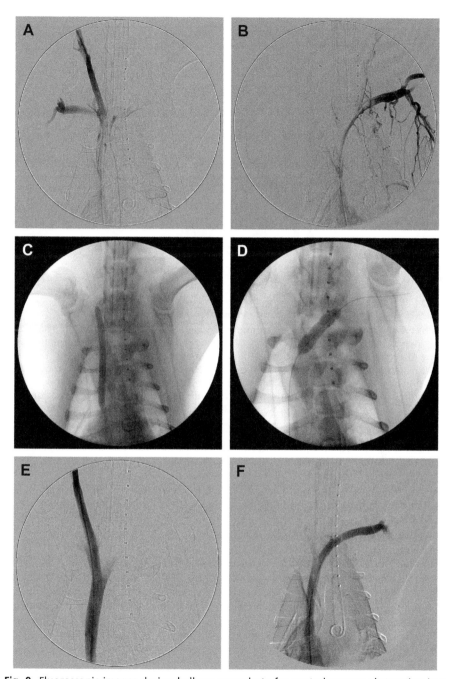

Fig. 9. Fluoroscopic images during balloon venoplasty for central venous obstruction in a dog. Thrombosis of the cranial vena cava as well as the right (*A*) and left (*B*) brachiocephalic veins developed after cardiopulmonary bypass surgery. Tissue plasminogen activator was infused throughout the thrombi, followed immediately by balloon venoplasty (*C*, *D*) to restore venous flow. The venograms of the right (*E*) and left (*F*) central veins demonstrated markedly improved flow and patency after this therapy. A pigtail marker catheter is present in the esophagus in all images for measurement calibration.

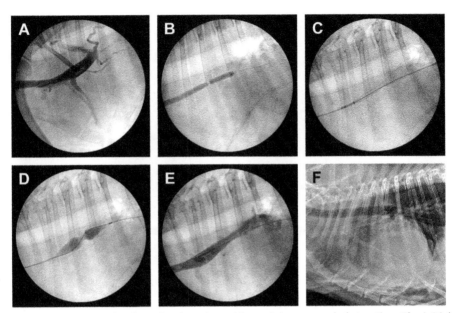

Fig. 10. Venous stent implantation in a dog with cranial vena caval obstruction. The initial venogram (*A*) demonstrates obstruction to venous return with collateral decompressing veins. After crossing the obstruction, a small high-pressure balloon is used to create a path for stent implantation (*B*). The stent is delivered across the obstruction (*C*) and further dilated by high-pressure balloon dilation (*D*). Improved venous return without collateral venous drainage is established at the procedure's end (*E*) with postoperative thoracic radiograph demonstrating final stent position (*F*). A pleural drainage catheter is also present in all images.

has been previously reported with survival of nearly 3 years in a dog after stent implantation.[62,63] In cases of luminal obstruction or extraluminal compression, self-expanding stents are preferred, as they continue to exert radial force after implantation. Sizing is determined relative to the adjacent lumen (eg, vena caval diameter) with a stent diameter chosen to be ~10% larger than the measured diameter. Stent length is determined by the distance that must be spanned to decompress the lesion. For transatrial stents, this distance stretches from caudal to cranial vena cava with at least 2 to 3 cm in each vessel to provide stent stability. Foreshortening must be considered at the time of stent placement, as well as the potential for additional foreshortening over time because the self-expanding stent will continue to exert radial force and may foreshorten further than observed at the time of implantation. In some cases, multiple stents may be placed coaxially to provide sufficient length to span the area of obstruction and provide purchase cranially and caudally (see **Fig. 11**).

EMBOLIC TRAPPING DEVICES

A vena cava filter is the most commonly used embolic trapping device in people. These devices are generally placed in the inferior vena cava to trap embolic particles originating from deep vein thrombosis, thus preventing pulmonary embolism. Superior vena cava filters have been placed to prevent pulmonary embolism in patients with upper extremity deep vein thrombosis. These devices have various shapes and range

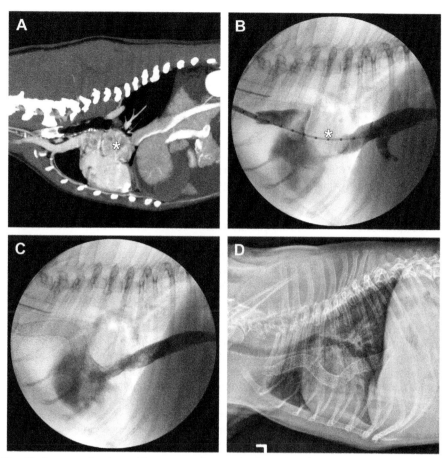

Fig. 11. Images of a dog with severe ascites and a large heart base mass obstructing the caudal vena cava undergoing transatrial stent implantation. The sagittal reformat maximal intensity projection computed tomography angiography image (*A*) shows the large mass (*asterisk*) resulting in near complete obstruction to caudal vena caval return. The angiogram before stent implantation (*B*) again demonstrates the filling defect of the mass (*asterisk*) with dilated hepatic veins and impaired caudal venous return. After 3 self-expanding stents are coaxially placed from cranial to caudal vena cava, the poststent angiogram (*C*) demonstrates absence of hepatic venous reflux and improved caudal venous return. The postoperative thoracic radiograph (*D*) illustrates final transatrial stent implantation.

from baskets to "spiderlike" endovascular conformations with the aim of trapping emboli before they reach the lung, allowing trapped emboli to undergo fibrinolysis (**Fig. 12**).

Filters are indicated in humans with a high risk of pulmonary embolism in whom anticoagulant therapy is contraindicated (severe thrombocytopenia, urgent surgery), patients with a massive clot burden, or in whom, despite anticoagulant therapy, pulmonary emboli have occurred. Despite their frequent use in people, few prospective studies have demonstrated survival benefit in patients.[64]

Filters can be inserted fluoroscopically into the vena cava via the jugular vein or femoral vein depending on the ease of access and the size of the patient. Filters

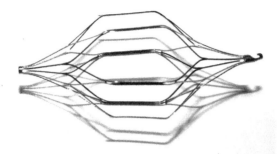

Fig. 12. A vena caval filter, designed for percutaneous placement in the inferior vena cava to capture thromboemboli from the inferior veins.

must be placed downstream from the thrombus. Filters can be made of nitinol or stainless steel and are biocompatible and nonthrombogenic (see **Fig. 12**). It is recommended to remove the filters once the underlying clot has been managed and they are provided with a retrieval wand that can be screwed onto or attached to the proximal aspect of the filter under fluoroscopy and pulled through a vascular sheath facilitating removal. Retrievability of filters has made these therapies a more attractive option for use in people.

In a literature review of caval filters in 11,000 patients, 65% were left in place and 35% were removed.[65] In filters that were not removed, reasons cited were need for a permanent indication in 21%, death in 19%, ongoing need for pulmonary embolism prevention in 19%, failed retrieval in 14%, loss to follow-up in 13%, physician oversight in 4%, and patient refusal in 3%. Approximately 90% of filters were successfully removed with a mean indwelling time of 106 days.[65] Some complications reported with filters include migration and tilting, fracture, embolization, penetration into the wall of the vena cava (19%, with 5% requiring a surgical intervention) and tearing or perforation of the cava at the time of placement.[64,65]

To the authors' knowledge, embolic filters have yet to be used in clinical veterinary patients for venous thrombosis. Possible indications in veterinary medicine could include dogs with adrenal neoplasia invading the caudal cava, or incidentally detected venous thrombosis in dogs with systemic disease likely to precipitate further thrombosis.[66] Preoperative placement of a vena cava filter in a dog with adrenal neoplasia may decrease the risk of pulmonary embolism during surgical resection.[67]

PORTAL VEIN OBSTRUCTION

Portal vein obstruction in veterinary medicine most commonly occurs secondary to thrombosis. Endothelial lesions causing portal hypertension, hypercoagulability, and/or sluggish portal flow may contribute to thrombus formation. Diseases associated with portal vein thrombosis in dogs include hepatic disease, neoplasia, immunologic disorders, hyperadrenocorticism, protein-losing enteropathy or nephropathy, and glucocorticoid administration.[68] In cats, portal vein thrombosis has been associated with hepatic disease and congenital portosystemic shunt.[69] Intraluminal or extraluminal neoplasia occurs less commonly, but can result in portal vein obstruction.

Given the unique anatomy of the portal vasculature, gaining access to the portal system, in the absence of a portosystemic shunt, is challenging. The portal vein arises caudal to the pancreas from the confluence of the cranial mesenteric and splenic veins. After entrance of the gastroduodenal vein, the portal vein then divides into a right and left branch just before entering the liver. Given its anatomy, thrombosis of the portal vein can occur with concomitant mesenteric and splenic vein thrombosis (**Figs. 13** and **14**). The goals of treating portal vein obstruction are to relieve clinical signs (ascites), prevent thrombus propagation, and prevent mesentery ischemia.

Little information on treatment and outcome of portal vein thrombosis exists in veterinary medicine. The following recommendations are based on the human medical literature and the authors' experience. Given the risk of bowel ischemia and poor liver perfusion, the requirement to treat portal vein thrombosis is usually immediate. Anticoagulants are administered, with LMWH (see **Table 2**) most commonly used in the authors' practice. Given the risk of bleeding and enterohepatic recirculation, the authors tend to avoid the use of warfarin. Direct oral Xa inhibitors may have decreased hepatic metabolism and, given the risk of gastrointestinal hemorrhage reported with these agents in dogs, as well as expense, they are not typically first-line therapy.

If the thrombus progresses despite adequate anticoagulation, thrombolysis and thrombectomy may be considered, although a hybrid surgical approach is likely required to access the portal vascular system. In people, transjugular intrahepatic shunt creation is used to relieve portal hypertension and provide a low-pressure run-off for portal flow. This procedure has yet to be reported in dogs and may be difficult to perform given the anatomy of the canine hepatic veins.[70]

Thrombolysis can be performed by administering tissue plasminogen activator or urokinase systemically, although direct delivery to the site of the thrombus is

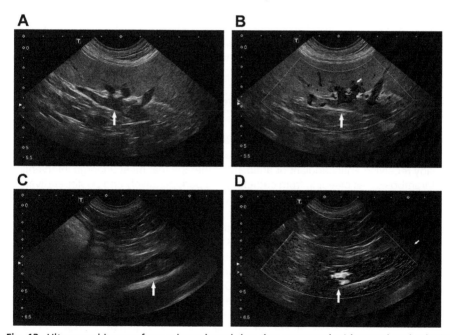

Fig. 13. Ultrasound images from a large-breed dog that presented with portal and splenic vein thrombosis. Marked congestion of the splenic vein and its branches with visible thrombus within the lumen (*arrow*) (*A*). Color flow Doppler shows lack of flow at the site of the thrombus (*large arrow*) and stagnant flow through congested splenic veins (*small arrow*) (*B*). A thrombus is visible in the portal vein (*arrow*) (*C*). Turbulent flow around the thrombus (*large arrow*) is seen on color flow Doppler with stagnant flow caudal to the portal vein thrombus (*small arrow*) (*D*).

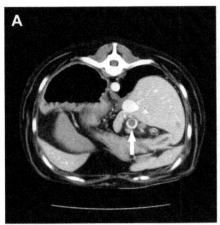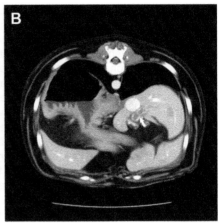

Fig. 14. Computed tomography angiography images from the same large-breed dog as in **Fig. 13.** A hypoattenuating filling defect (*arrow*) is visible in the portal vein (*A*). Thrombus can also be seen extending into the splenic vein (*arrow*) (*B*).

preferable. Infusion of thrombolytic agents directly into the mesenteric artery via femoral or radial arterial access has been reported in people to achieve higher concentrations of the thrombolytic agent in the portal vein, but has not been evaluated in dogs.[71] In small animals, access to the cranial mesenteric artery can be achieved either by femoral or carotid arterial access, depending on patient size. Open surgical thrombectomy of portal vein thrombosis also may be considered and may allow for a hybrid approach to management with direct catheterization of the portal vasculature.

PREOPERATIVE, PERIOPERATIVE, AND POSTOPERATIVE MANAGEMENT OF ANTITHROMBOTIC MEDICATIONS

Before, during, and after thrombosis intervention, the question of medical anticoagulation becomes important. How should medication schedules be altered in patients already receiving anticoagulant or antiplatelet therapy that must undergo intervention for thrombosis? As bleeding from catheter sites perioperatively and postoperatively is a concern, discontinuation of anticoagulant and antiplatelet therapy before a procedure is often considered. The length of time required for discontinuation of therapy is variable and dependent on the half-life of the agent being given. Based on the short half-life of unfractionated heparin, it can be stopped 2 to 5 hours before a procedure. Given the longer half-life of LMWH or direct Xa inhibitors, these should be stopped 8 hours before a procedure.[31,72,73] Aspirin causes irreversible platelet inactivation by irreversibly binding cyclooxygenase. Despite its antiplatelet properties, clinical bleeding with aspirin therapy appears to be uncommon.[74] Clopidogrel is a potent antiplatelet medication, and complications in people undergoing interventional procedures have been reported. It should therefore be discontinued 7 days before a procedure.[75]

Despite these recommendations, in an emergency situation, an intervention can be performed despite concurrent anticoagulant/antiplatelet therapy. The clinician must be prepared for bleeding complications and, if needed, may be able to reverse the effects of heparin with the use of protamine or by transfusion of activated clotting factors in the case of LMWH.[76]

Following thrombosis intervention, decisions about continued antithrombotic therapy are also important. If the underlying disease that predisposed to thrombus formation is not addressed, the patient may thrombose other sites or present with recurrence at the same site. In people, many factors are taken into account, such as underlying disease, site of the thrombus, and site of the implant, if present, when determining an adequate anticoagulant protocol.[74]

There is very little information in the veterinary literature on whether to continue anticoagulant and/or antiplatelet medication postoperatively. According to human recommendations, the presence of a vascular stent does not augment thrombogenesis, but anticoagulant/antiplatelet medication should be continued as long as the underlying disease that led to thrombosis is present.[74]

In veterinary medicine, decisions on long-term anticoagulant and antiplatelet therapy are often chosen with regard to ease of administration and cost, with limited evidence to guide optimal therapy.

SUMMARY

Vascular obstructions in small animals have numerous etiologies and variable clinical signs depending on location and chronicity. Once identified, a decision must be made whether or not to intervene and which therapeutic method is most appropriate (medical, interventional, or surgical). A combined approach of angioplasty, vascular stenting, or catheter-directed thrombolysis may be most appropriate for acute thrombosis, although optimal therapeutic strategies are undefined in this population. Percutaneous mechanical thrombectomy, if available, also may be appropriate. The role of embolic trapping devices in animals is uncertain, but these devices may prove useful for cases of chronic venous thrombosis to limit pulmonary emboli. More chronic cases of vascular obstruction, in whom collateral pathways have developed and neither ischemia nor venous congestion are manifest, may be managed by conservative medical therapies. Prospective clinical studies are needed to better guide our management of vascular obstructions in veterinary medicine.

REFERENCES

1. Dunn M. Acquired coagulopathies. In: Ettinger SJ, Feldman BF, editors. Textbook of veterinary internal medicine, vol. 1, 7th edition. Philadelphia: Elsevier; 2010. p. 797–801.
2. Montoro-Garcia S, Schindewolf M, Stanford S, et al. The role of platelets in venous thromboembolism. Semin Thromb Hemost 2016;42(3):242–51.
3. Dunn ME. Thrombectomy and thrombolysis: the interventional radiology approach. J Vet Emerg Crit Care (San Antonio) 2011;21(2):144–50.
4. Dunn ME, Weisse C. Thrombectomy and thrombolysis. In: Weisse C, Berent A, editors. Veterinary image-guided interventions. John Wiley & Sons, Ltd; 2015. p. 464–78.
5. Hogan DF. Feline cardiogenic arterial thromboembolism: prevention and therapy. Vet Clin North Am Small Anim Pract 2017;47(5):1065–82.
6. Smith SA, Tobias AH, Jacob KA, et al. Arterial thromboembolism in cats: acute crisis in 127 cases (1992-2001) and long-term management with low-dose aspirin in 24 cases. J Vet Intern Med 2003;17(1):73–83.
7. Winter RL, Sedacca CD, Adams A, et al. Aortic thrombosis in dogs: presentation, therapy, and outcome in 26 cases. J Vet Cardiol 2012;14(2):333–42.

8. Guillaumin J, Hmelo S, Farrell K, et al. Canine aortic thromboembolism (2005-2011): a retrospective study of 50 cases. J Vet Emerg Crit Care (San Antonio) 2012;22(S2):S6.

9. Lake-Bakaar GA, Johnson EG, Griffiths LG. Aortic thrombosis in dogs: 31 cases (2000-2010). J Am Vet Med Assoc 2012;241(7):910–5.

10. Williams TP, Shaw S, Porter A, et al. Aortic thrombosis in dogs. J Vet Emerg Crit Care (San Antonio) 2017;27(1):9–22.

11. Winter RL, Budke CM. Multicenter evaluation of signalment and comorbid conditions associated with aortic thrombotic disease in dogs. J Am Vet Med Assoc 2017;251(4):438–42.

12. Ahmed S, Raman SP, Fishman EK. CT angiography and 3D imaging in aortoiliac occlusive disease: collateral pathways in Leriche syndrome. Abdom Radiol (NY) 2017;42(9):2346–57.

13. Waldrop JE, Stoneham AE, Tidwell AS, et al. Aortic dissection associated with aortic aneurysms and posterior paresis in a dog. J Vet Intern Med 2003;17(2):223–9.

14. Ranck RS, Linder KE, Haber MD, et al. Primary intimal aortic angiosarcoma in a dog. Vet Pathol 2008;45(3):361–4.

15. Kohnken R, Durham JA, Premanandan C, et al. Aortic chondroid neoplasia in two Labrador retriever dogs. J Vet Cardiol 2015;17(4):314–20.

16. Laste NJ, Harpster NK. A retrospective study of 100 cases of feline distal aortic thromboembolism—1977-1993. J Am Anim Hosp Assoc 1995;31(6):492–500.

17. Guillaumin J, Goy-Thollot I, Bonagura J. Thrombolysis with tissue plasminogen activator (TPA) in feline acute aortic thromboembolism: 19 cases (2011-2015). J Vet Emerg Crit Care (San Antonio) 2015;25(S1):S13.

18. Reimer SB, Kittleson MD, Kyles AE. Use of rheolytic thrombectomy in the treatment of feline distal aortic thromboembolism. J Vet Intern Med 2006;20(2):290–6.

19. Scott KC, Hansen BD, DeFrancesco TC. Coagulation effects of low molecular weight heparin compared with heparin in dogs considered to be at risk for clinically significant venous thrombosis. J Vet Emerg Crit Care (San Antonio) 2009;19(1):74–80.

20. Weitz JI. Low-molecular-weight heparins. N Engl J Med 1997;337(10):688–98.

21. Smith CE, Rozanski EA, Freeman LM, et al. Use of low molecular weight heparin in cats: 57 cases (1999-2003). J Am Vet Med Assoc 2004;225(8):1237–41.

22. Smith S, Tobias A. Feline arterial thromboembolism: an update. Vet Clin North Am Small Anim Pract 2004;34(5):1245–71.

23. Lynch AM, deLaforcade AM, Sharp CR. Clinical experience of anti-Xa monitoring in critically ill dogs receiving dalteparin. J Vet Emerg Crit Care (San Antonio) 2014;24(4):421–8.

24. Alwood AJ, Downend AB, Brooks MB, et al. Anticoagulant effects of low-molecular-weight heparins in healthy cats. J Vet Intern Med 2007;21(3):378–87.

25. Van De Wiele CM, Hogan DF, Green HW, et al. Antithrombotic effect of enoxaparin in clinically healthy cats: a venous stasis model. J Vet Intern Med 2010;24(1):185–91.

26. Connolly SJ, Ezekowitz MD, Yusuf S, et al. Dabigatran versus warfarin in patients with atrial fibrillation. N Engl J Med 2009;361(12):1139–51.

27. Patel MR, Mahaffey KW, Garg J, et al. Rivaroxaban versus warfarin in nonvalvular atrial fibrillation. N Engl J Med 2011;365(10):883–91.

28. Granger CB, Alexander JH, McMurray JJ, et al. Apixaban versus warfarin in patients with atrial fibrillation. N Engl J Med 2011;365(11):981–92.

29. Yang VK, Cunningham SM, Rush JE, et al. The use of rivaroxaban for the treatment of thrombotic complications in four dogs. J Vet Emerg Crit Care (San Antonio) 2016;26(5):729–36.
30. Morassi A, Bianco D, Park E, et al. Evaluation of the safety and tolerability of rivaroxaban in dogs with presumed primary immune-mediated hemolytic anemia. J Vet Emerg Crit Care (San Antonio) 2016;26(4):488–94.
31. Conversy B, Blais MC, Dunn M, et al. Anticoagulant activity of oral rivaroxaban in healthy dogs. Vet J 2017;223:5–11.
32. Dixon-Jimenez AC, Brainard BM, Brooks MB, et al. Pharmacokinetic and pharmacodynamic evaluation of oral rivaroxaban in healthy adult cats. J Vet Emerg Crit Care (San Antonio) 2016;26(5):619–29.
33. Myers JA, Wittenburg LA, Olver CS, et al. Pharmacokinetics and pharmacodynamics of the factor Xa inhibitor apixaban after oral and intravenous administration to cats. Am J Vet Res 2015;76(8):732–8.
34. Specchi S, d'Anjou MA, Carmel EN, et al. Computed tomographic characteristics of collateral venous pathways in dogs with caudal vena cava obstruction. Vet Radiol Ultrasound 2014;55(5):531–8.
35. Ricciardi M, Lanci M. Acquired collateral venous pathways in a dog with cranial vena cava obstruction. J Vet Med Sci 2017;79(11):1772–5.
36. Montavon PM, Arnold P, von Segesser LK. Chronic peritoneal effusion secondary to partial caudal vena cava obstruction following traumatic pneumothorax in a dog. Vet Comp Orthop Traumatol 2007;20(4):340–5.
37. Taylor S, Rozanski E, Sato AF, et al. Vascular stent placement for palliation of mass-associated chylothorax in two dogs. J Am Vet Med Assoc 2017;251(6):696–701.
38. Malik R, Hunt GB, Chard RB, et al. Congenital obstruction of the caudal vena cava in a dog. J Am Vet Med Assoc 1990;197(7):880–2.
39. Macintire DK, Henderson RH, Banfield C, et al. Budd-Chiari syndrome in a kitten, caused by membranous obstruction of the caudal vena cava. J Am Anim Hosp Assoc 1995;31(6):484–91.
40. Hoehne SN, Milovancev M, Hyde AJ, et al. Placement of a caudal vena cava stent for treatment of Budd-Chiari-like syndrome in a 4-month-old Ragdoll cat. J Am Vet Med Assoc 2014;245(4):414–8.
41. Van De Wiele CM, Hogan DF, Green HW 3rd, et al. Cranial vena caval syndrome secondary to transvenous pacemaker implantation in two dogs. J Vet Cardiol 2008;10(2):155–61.
42. Stauthammer C, Tobias A, France M, et al. Caudal vena cava obstruction caused by redundant pacemaker lead in a dog. J Vet Cardiol 2009;11(2):141–5.
43. Mulz JM, Kraus MS, Thompson M, et al. Cranial vena caval syndrome secondary to central venous obstruction associated with a pacemaker lead in a dog. J Vet Cardiol 2010;12(3):217–23.
44. Pelosi A, Prinsen JK, Eyster GE, et al. Caudal vena cava kinking in dogs with ascites. Vet Radiol Ultrasound 2012;53(3):233–5.
45. Lisciandro GR, Harvey HJ, Beck KA. Automobile-induced obstruction of the intrathoracic caudal vena cava in a dog. J Small Anim Pract 1995;36(8):368–72.
46. Fine DM, Olivier NB, Walshaw R, et al. Surgical correction of late-onset Budd-Chiari-like syndrome in a dog. J Am Vet Med Assoc 1998;212(6):835–7.
47. Howard J, Arceneaux KA, Paugh-Partington B, et al. Blastomycosis granuloma involving the cranial vena cava associated with chylothorax and cranial vena caval syndrome in a dog. J Am Anim Hosp Assoc 2000;36(2):159–61.

48. Font A, Closa JM. Ultrasonographic localization of a caudal vena cava thrombus in a dog with leishmaniasis. Vet Radiol Ultrasound 1997;38(5):394–6.

49. LeGrange SN, Fossum TW, Lemire T, et al. Thrombosis of the caudal vena cava presenting as an unusual cause of an abdominal mass and thrombocytopenia in a dog. J Am Anim Hosp Assoc 2000;36(2):143–51.

50. Saridomichelakis MN, Koutinas CK, Souftas V, et al. Extensive caudal vena cava thrombosis secondary to unilateral renal tubular cell carcinoma in a dog. J Small Anim Pract 2004;45(2):108–12.

51. Schoeman JP, Stidworthy MF. Budd-Chiari-like syndrome associated with an adrenal phaeochromocytoma in a dog. J Small Anim Pract 2001;42(4):191–4.

52. Wey AC, Moore FM. Right atrial chromaffin paraganglioma in a dog. J Vet Cardiol 2012;14(3):459–64.

53. Adin DB, Thomas WP. Balloon dilation of cor triatriatum dexter in a dog. J Vet Intern Med 1999;13(6):617–9.

54. Atkins C, DeFrancesco T. Balloon dilation of cor triatriatum dexter in a dog. J Vet Intern Med 2000;14(5):471–2.

55. Schrope DP. Hepatic vein stenosis (Budd-Chiari syndrome) as a cause of ascites in a cat. J Vet Cardiol 2010;12(3):197–202.

56. Leblanc N, Defrancesco TC, Adams AK, et al. Cutting balloon catheterization for interventional treatment of cor triatriatum dexter: 2 cases. J Vet Cardiol 2012; 14(4):525–30.

57. Haskal ZJ, Dumbleton SA, Holt D. Percutaneous treatment of caval obstruction and Budd-Chiari syndrome in a cat. J Vasc Interv Radiol 1999;10(4):487–9.

58. Barncord K, Stauthammer C, Moen SL, et al. Stent placement for palliation of cor triatriatum dexter in a dog with suspected patent foramen ovale. J Vet Cardiol 2016;18(1):79–87.

59. Scansen BA. Interventional cardiology: what's new? Vet Clin North Am Small Anim Pract 2017;47(5):1021–40.

60. Horikawa M, Quencer KB. Central venous interventions. Tech Vasc Interv Radiol 2017;20(1):48–57.

61. Fleck D, Albadawi H, Shamoun F, et al. Catheter-directed thrombolysis of deep vein thrombosis: literature review and practice considerations. Cardiovasc Diagn Ther 2017;7(Suppl 3):s228–37.

62. Weisse C, Berent A, Scansen BA, et al. Transatrial stenting for long-term management of tumor obstruction of the right atrium in 3 dogs. Vet Surg 2012;42:E112.

63. Weisse C, Scansen BA. Cardiac tumor palliation. In: Weisse C, Berent A, editors. Veterinary image-guided interventions. John Wiley & Sons, Ltd; 2015. p. 556–63.

64. Duffett L, Carrier M. Inferior vena cava filters. J Thromb Haemost 2017;15(1): 3–12.

65. Jia Z, Fuller TA, McKinney JM, et al. Utility of retrievable inferior vena cava filters: a systematic literature review and analysis of the reasons for nonretrieval of filters with temporary indications. Cardiovasc Intervent Radiol 2018. https://doi.org/10. 1007/s00270-018-1880-9.

66. Barrera JS, Bernard F, Ehrhart EJ, et al. Evaluation of risk factors for outcome associated with adrenal gland tumors with or without invasion of the caudal vena cava and treated via adrenalectomy in dogs: 86 cases (1993-2009). J Am Vet Med Assoc 2013;242(12):1715–21.

67. Massari F, Nicoli S, Romanelli G, et al. Adrenalectomy in dogs with adrenal gland tumors: 52 cases (2002-2008). J Am Vet Med Assoc 2011;239(2):216–21.

68. Respess M, O'Toole TE, Taeymans O, et al. Portal vein thrombosis in 33 dogs: 1998-2011. J Vet Intern Med 2012;26(2):230–7.

69. Rogers CL, O'Toole TE, Keating JH, et al. Portal vein thrombosis in cats: 6 cases (2001-2006). J Vet Intern Med 2008;22(2):282–7.
70. Levien AS, Weisse C, Donovan TA, et al. Assessment of the efficacy and potential complications of transjugular liver biopsy in canine cadavers. J Vet Intern Med 2014;28(2):338–45.
71. Liu FY, Wang MQ, Fan QS, et al. Interventional treatment for symptomatic acute-subacute portal and superior mesenteric vein thrombosis. World J Gastroenterol 2009;15(40):5028–34.
72. Mischke RH, Schuttert C, Grebe SI. Anticoagulant effects of repeated subcutaneous injections of high doses of unfractionated heparin in healthy dogs. Am J Vet Res 2001;62(12):1887–91.
73. Grebe S, Jacobs C, Kietzmann M, et al. Phamacokinetics of low-molecular-weight heparins Fragmin D in dogs. Berl Munch Tierarztl Wochenschr 2000;113(3): 103–7 [in German].
74. Mehta RP, Johnson MS. Update on anticoagulant medications for the interventional radiologist. J Vasc Interv Radiol 2006;17(4):597–612.
75. Hogan DF, Andrews DA, Green HW, et al. Antiplatelet effects and pharmacodynamics of clopidogrel in cats. J Am Vet Med Assoc 2004;225(9):1406–11.
76. Dunn M, Brooks MB. Antiplatelet and anticoagulant therapy. In: Bonagura JD, Twedt DC, editors. Current veterinary therapy XIV. Philadelphia: Saunders; 2009. p. 24–8.

Interventional Radiology and Interventional Endoscopy in Treatment of Nephroureteral Disease in the Dog and Cat

Alexander Gallagher, DVM, MS

KEYWORDS

- Ureteral obstruction • Ureteral stent • Subcutaneous ureteral bypass
- Ectopic ureter • Idiopathic renal hematuria • Laser ablation

KEY POINTS

- Interventional endoscopy and interventional radiology allow for minimally invasive techniques in the treatment of kidney and ureteral disease in the dog and cat.
- Ureteral obstructions are being diagnosed with increased frequency in veterinary medicine and may lead to the development of obstructive nephropathy, pyonephrosis, and critical illness.
- Prompt recognition and treatment of ureteral obstructions is needed to provide the best return of renal function.
- Renal pelvic dilation greater than 13 mm is consistent with ureteral obstruction, but smaller dilations may also be caused by obstruction and require antegrade pyelography to further access.

INTRODUCTION

Dogs and cats are commonly affected by diseases of the kidneys and ureters. In the past, many of these diseases were only treatable with invasive surgeries or may not have had a treatment option. In recent years, advancements in equipment and techniques has allowed the development of minimally invasive urology procedures, alone or combined with surgery, to treat many conditions of the urinary tract. These techniques rely on imaging including fluoroscopy, ultrasound, and endoscopy, often in combination. This article focuses on the current evidence for application of minimally invasive endourologic procedures for management of diseases of the kidney and ureter.

Disclosure Statement: The author has nothing to disclose.
Small Animal Medicine, Department of Small Animal Clinical Sciences, College of Veterinary Medicine, University of Florida, 2015 Southwest 16th Avenue, Gainesville, FL 32608, USA
E-mail address: gallaghera@ufl.edu

KIDNEY
Idiopathic Renal Hematuria

Idiopathic renal hematuria (IRH) is a rare condition in dogs with only 27 cases reported in the literature.[1-10] It is characterized by chronic, often gross, hematuria that is not associated with hematologic or radiologic abnormalities. Bleeding can lead to the formation of clots in the renal pelvis, ureter, or bladder with possible obstruction of the urinary tract.[1,3] Most cases occur in young, large breed dogs, but it has also been reported in older dogs and smaller breeds.[7] Of the 27 reported cases, 19 (70%) were unilateral, seven (26%) were bilateral (three of these dogs were initially unilateral), and one was undetermined if unilateral or bilateral. In addition, IRH has been anecdotally reported in cats.[11]

Diagnosis of IRH requires visualization of the urine jets at the ureterovesicular junction (UVJ), most commonly by cystoscopy (**Fig. 1**D). Bright red blood is typically seen from the side that is bleeding. Because of the intermittent bleeding in some cases, cystoscopy may reveal grossly normal urine jets if there is not active bleeding at the time of cystoscopy. In these cases, cystoscopy should be repeated as soon as the owner notes return of gross hematuria. In people, strenuous exercise (eg, climbing stairs) before cystoscopy has been recommended to improve the likelihood of detecting bleeding in patients without gross hematuria.[12] Cystotomy with ureteral catheterization can also be done, but care must be used to prevent iatrogenic trauma and bleeding from the ureters during catheterization.

Previously, IRH has been treated by nephrectomy in cases with unilateral bleeding.[1-3] In one dog with unilateral IRH, manual compression of the dorsal ramus of the renal artery resulted in cessation of hematuria intraoperatively. Subsequently, the dorsal ramus was ligated with resolution of gross hematuria.[4] Because greater than 25% of cases are bilateral and lesions are likely not parenchymal, renal-sparing techniques as used in people including sclerotherapy and ureteroscopy with cauterization have been investigated to avoid nephrectomy.

Sclerotherapy

Sclerotherapy involves the instillation of cauterizing agents into the renal pelvis and has recently been reported as a successful renal-sparing technique for treatment of IRH in dogs.[7-10] Under endoscopic and fluoroscopic guidance, a ureteral catheter, with or without an occlusion balloon, is placed and the sclerosing agents infused into the affected renal pelvis. After the procedure, a ureteral stent is placed to prevent ureteral obstruction caused by ureteritis that may occur secondary to the sclerosing agents (**Fig. 1**). Commonly used agents in dogs include silver nitrate and/or povidone-iodine.

Berent and colleagues[7] initially described an endoscopic-guided technique using a combination of both agents in six dogs, five male and one female. Initially, one dog had bilateral hematuria and five had unilateral hematuria. One dog developed hematuria on the contralateral side 4.5 months after sclerotherapy for a total of eight renal pelvises treated. Complete resolution of gross hematuria occurred in five of six dogs (six of eight renal pelvises) within 1 week (median, 6 hours; range, 0–7 days). All dogs had resolution of anemia, pollakiuria, and stranguria. Since this study, Berent[13] has reported performing sclerotherapy in greater than 25 dogs with a success rate of 80% to 85% including success in one dog treated with povidone-iodine alone.

Di Cicco and colleagues[8] reported on a dog with IRH treated with silver nitrate alone. At cystotomy, urine from the right ureter was grossly normal but had microscopic hematuria. Urine from the left ureter was grossly hematuric. Silver nitrate was instilled in the left renal pelvis. The urine was grossly normal at discharge from

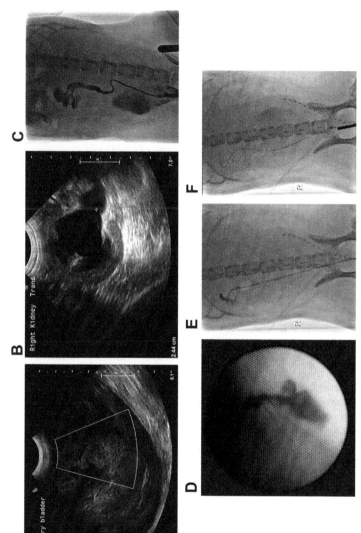

Fig. 1. Sclerotherapy for treatment of idiopathic renal hematuria in a dog. (*A*) A large, echogenic, nonvascular mass is noted in the bladder consistent with a blood clot on ultrasound imaging. (*B*) Transverse ultrasound image of the right kidney shows severe hydronephrosis. An echogenic mass was seen in the proximal ureter consistent with a blood clot (not pictured). (*C*) A retrograde contrast pyeloureterogram shows hydronephrosis and proximal hydroureter. A filling defect is noted at the ureteropelvic junction consistent with a blood clot. A ureteral stent was placed to allow drainage of the kidney pending sclerotherapy (not shown). (*D*) Hematuria noted from the right ureterovesicular junction during cystoscopy. (*E*) During sclerotherapy 1 week later, a retrograde pyeloureterogram was repeated with a balloon catheter present near the ureteropelvic junction to measure the volume of the renal pelvis. Notice the marked improvement in hydronephrosis and hydroureter. (*F*) After the sclerotherapy, a ureteral stent is placed to prevent ureteral obstruction.

the hospital. Ten months later the dog developed gross hematuria and surgical instillation of silver nitrate in the left renal pelvis was repeated but bleeding continued. A left nephrectomy was performed, but 2 days after surgery severe hematuria recurred with suspected obstruction of the right kidney caused by blood clot and the dog was euthanized.

Most recently, Adelman and colleagues[9] reported the use of povidone-iodine alone for the treatment of unilateral IRH in two dogs. The first dog had resolution of gross hematuria within 24 hours of sclerotherapy. At recheck 4 months later, the owner reported no gross hematuria, although urinalysis revealed mild microscopic hematuria. The second dog also had resolution of gross hematuria within 24 hours. No gross hematuria was noted at 14 days post-procedure, but microscopic hematuria was present. Two months after sclerotherapy the owners reported no evidence of gross hematuria.

Complications associated with sclerotherapy have included flank pain, ureteritis, and ureteral obstruction. These may be associated with leakage of sclerosing agents from the renal pelvis into the ureter. Because of this risk, ureteral stenting at the time of sclerotherapy is recommended. Because of increased risk of stent migration, removal of the stent is recommended in 2 to 4 weeks.[7] Sclerotherapy seems to be a successful renal-sparing technique for treatment of IRH.

Ureteroscopy

Ureteroscopy with cauterization is the treatment of choice for chronic unilateral hematuria in people. Despite advances in scope technology, ureteroscopy in the dog is still limited because of the small diameter of the canine ureter (0.5–2.0 mm). It is typically reserved for dogs greater than 20 kg or when a ureteral stent has been previously placed for 1 to 2 weeks to create passive dilation of the ureter. If a bleeding lesion is identified, it is cauterized with a Bugbee cautery probe or by holmium:YAG laser.[14] The success rate of ureteroscopy with cauterization has not been reported in dogs.

URETER

Obstruction of the ureter, particularly in cats, is increasing in veterinary medicine.[15,16] This may be caused by a true increase in incidence or by better recognition of the condition. The pathophysiology of ureteral obstruction is complex and likely differs between species.[17] Several experimental models of complete and partial obstruction in dogs have been reported with varying results.[18–23]

Kerr[18,19] studied a complete unilateral obstruction model in dogs by ligating the ureter for periods of 7, 14, 21, or 28 days. Immediately after removal of the obstructive ureteral ligature, the mean glomerular filtration rates (GFR) as a percent of the preligation value were 27% and 4% for 7 and 14 days, respectively. For dogs ligated for 21 and 28 days (one each), initial GFR could not be obtained until Days 18 and 23 postligature removal, at which time GFR was 33% and 13%, respectively. Time to maximum recovery was 4 to 57 days (mean, 22 days) with a mean final GFR of 68% for the 7-day group, 62 days with GFR 39% in the 14-day dog, 28 days with GFR 37% in 21-day dog, and 30 days with GFR 22% in 28-day dog.

In the same studies,[18,19] nephrectomy of the contralateral kidney was performed 5 days after removal of the obstructive ureteral ligature in two dogs of the 7-day group, and one dog each in the 14-, 21-, and 28-day group. Four to 5 days postremoval, percent of preligation GFR was 160% and 89% for two dogs in 7-day group, 54% for 14-day dog, 46% for 21-day dog, and 53% for 28-day dog. Days to maximum recovery (percent GFR) for each group were 5 days (140%) and 12 days (180%); 17 days (114%); 19 days (108%); and 22 days (95%).

Vaughan and Gillenwater[20] performed similar studies in dogs after 7, 14, 28, 42, and 56 days of unilateral obstruction. Results for dogs in the 7-, 14-, and 28-day groups were similar to previous studies. In dogs ligated for 42 or 56 days, there was no return of function by 1 month after removal of the ligature. Pelvic volumes were measured at the time of ureter release and ranged from 23 mL in the 7-day group to 140 mL in the 56-day group. Following recovery, there was marked reduction in the pelvic capacity to less than 10 mL in all dogs, even in the 56-day group.

Fink and colleagues[22] evaluated the degree of recovery after unilateral ureteral obstruction for 4, 7, and 21 days. Recovery for the 7- and 21-day groups was similar to that reported by Kerr and Vaughan. For dogs in the 4-day group, recovery was nearly complete with a mean GFR 93% of preligation at 3 to 4 weeks. Additionally, five dogs had ligation of 14 days followed by contralateral nephrectomy at 12 weeks postopening of the ureter. Before nephrectomy, GFR was 53% of preligation and improved to 127% 12 to 20 weeks afterward.

Lastly, Leahy and colleagues[23] evaluated recovery in dogs after 14, 28, or 60 days of partial ureteral obstruction followed by neoureterocystostomy. All dogs in the 14-day group recovered normal function, whereas dogs in the 28-day and 60-day groups recovered 31% and 8%, respectively, of normal function after 28 days. Both of these latter groups were noted to be anuric at the time of neoureterocystostomy.

Based on these findings, early intervention to relieve obstruction seems critical to maximize recovery of renal function. Ideally, acute complete obstructions should be resolved within 4 days and partial obstructions within 14 days. Studies in cats have not been performed and it is unknown how recovery in this species compares with dogs. The dogs in the experimental models likely had normal kidneys before ureteral obstruction, whereas many of the animals with ureteral obstruction likely have some degree of underlying chronic kidney disease (CKD). Hence, preservation of all function should be a priority, because the baseline number of functional nephrons may be reduced before the initiation of the acute obstructive insult.

The improvement in GFR of obstructed kidneys after contralateral nephrectomy of a normal kidney is interesting. This finding suggests that there may be functional reserve present in the kidneys even after extended recovery periods. In animals with CKD where the contralateral kidney has decreased compensatory function, return of function in the obstructed kidney may be greater even after prolonged obstruction. Treatment of these kidneys regardless of duration of obstruction may be warranted, although further studies are needed to assess efficacy.

Benign Ureteral Obstructions

Ureteral obstruction is most often cause by ureterolithiasis, with other causes including congenital or acquired strictures, iatrogenic ligation, trauma, and solidified blood calculi.[15,24–29] Calcium-containing stones are present in 98% of cats and greater than 50% of dogs preventing medical dissolution from being used in most cases.[15,16,30] Additionally, given the negative consequences of ureteral obstruction on renal function, medical dissolution should not be attempted in cases of obstructive nephropathy secondary to ureterolithiasis.

Diagnosis of ureteral obstruction often relies on routine imaging, including abdominal radiographs and abdominal ultrasound. In a study of 11 cats with ureteral obstruction, sensitivity of radiographs (based on presence of ureteral calculi) and ultrasound to identify obstruction was 60% and 100%, and specificity was 100% and 30%, respectively.[31] Antegrade pyelography was found to be 100% sensitive and specific. In a larger study of 101 cats with ureteral calculi, sensitivity of radiographs alone was

81%, ultrasound alone was 77%, and combined imaging was 90% to determine the presence of ureteroliths.[16]

Ultrasonographic findings of renal pelvic dilation concurrent with ureteral dilation secondary to a known obstructive lesion is considered diagnostic for ureteral obstruction.[13] However, in some cases, such as strictures or solidified blood clots, a specific lesion within the ureter may not be seen. Renal pelvic and ureteral dilation is seen with other processes, such as diuresis, pyelonephritis, CKD, and ectopic ureter (EU) resulting in a diagnostic dilemma. Several studies have evaluated ultrasound findings to determine if the degree of renal pelvic or ureteral dilation can predict obstruction.

D'Anjou and colleagues[32] evaluated 81 dogs and 66 cats with sonographically diagnosed renal pelvic dilation. The maximal pelvic width was compared between animals with normal renal function (with or without diuresis) and those with nonobstructive urinary disease and those with obstruction. They found that pelvic widths overlapped among all groups, but a width greater than 13 mm in cats and dogs was only found in obstructive disease where median (range) pelvic width was 15.1 mm (5.1–76.2 mm) in dogs and 6.8 mm (1.2–39.1 mm) in cats. In another study, sonographic features of 37 cats with 45 obstructed ureters confirmed by pyelography were described.[33] Median (range) pelvic height was 6.9 mm (0–37 mm) with 24% measuring less than 4 mm and two ureters less than 2 mm. Median ureteral diameter was 3.2 mm (0–11 mm) with 27% of ureters less than 2 mm. Ureteral stones were seen in 64% of ureters.

Most recently, Quimby and colleagues[34] evaluated renal pelvic and ureteral measurements in normal cats (n = 10) and cats with CKD (n = 66), pyelonephritis (n = 13), or ureteral obstruction (n = 11, confirmed by surgery). Cats with ureteral obstructions had renal pelvic heights greater than normal and CKD cats, but not cats with pyelonephritis. Similar to D'Anjou and coworkers,[32] renal pelvic height greater than 13 mm was attributable to ureteral obstruction. Median (range) greatest pelvic height in obstructed cats was 10.4 mm (3.1–19.3 mm). Ureteral dilation was present in 6% of CKD cats, 46% of pyelonephritis cats, and 82% of ureteral obstructions. Cats with ureteral obstruction had ureteral dilation greater than normal and CKD cats, but not cats with pyelonephritis. No cats with CKD or pyelonephritis had a ureteral dilation greater than 5.3 mm, whereas more than 75% of cats with ureteral obstruction had a dilation greater than 6 mm.

Based on these findings, renal pelvic height greater than 13 mm in cats and dogs is consistent with obstruction, even if a specific lesion is not seen on imaging. In cats, a ureteral diameter greater than 6 mm is likely consistent with obstruction. Of particular note, obstructions in cats may be associated with minimal renal pelvic or ureteral distention. In cases where routine imaging is inconclusive and ureteral obstruction is still a concern, antegrade pyelography should be performed. Antegrade pyelography allows better visualization of the renal pelvis and ureters than excretory urography, especially in cases of complete obstruction. In addition, it reduces the risk of contrast-induced kidney injury. Potential complications include renal hemorrhage, renal pelvic laceration, and renal pelvic clot formation. Leakage of contrast from the pelvis can occur and may result in a poor or nondiagnostic study.[35]

Treatment options include medical management, surgery, and placement of stents or subcutaneous ureteral bypass devices (SUBs). Medical management may consist of intravenous fluids, diuretics, pain medications, and α_1-antagonists. In one study, 52 cats were treated with medical management alone for ureteral calculi.[15] Seven cats (13%) responded based on decreases in creatinine concentration. In four out of seven cats, follow-up radiographs showed passage of the ureterolith into the bladder. Serial imaging was performed in seven cats with no change in creatinine and showed passage of the ureteral stone into the bladder in five cats. Although the success rate is low, medical management should be considered for 24 hours, unless otherwise contraindicated, because of risks involved with other interventions.

Traditional surgical techniques include ureterotomy, neoureterocystostomy, and ureteronephrectomy. In a small study, 16 dogs underwent surgery for ureteral calculi.[36] Perioperative mortality was 6.25% and 14% had recurrent obstruction within 30 days. Ten of 16 dogs (63%) had azotemia initially and 6 of 14 (43%) were azotemic postoperatively, including one dog that was initially nonazotemic. An early study of ureteral surgery in cats showed 31% had postoperative complications and a mortality rate of 18%.[15] Fifty-six of 71 cats (79%) were initially azotemic and 31 of 71 (44%) were azotemic at discharge. Roberts and colleagues[37] and Culp and colleagues[38] have reported similar perioperative mortality rate of 21% and 22%, respectively. However, Wormser and colleagues[39] recently reported a much lower mortality rate of 8%.

Because of the reported morbidity and mortality associated with ureteral surgery and low success rate of medical management in the cat, other treatment modalities have been investigated including nephrostomy tubes, ureteral stents, and SUBs. Nephrostomy tubes are mainly used for short-term stabilization of animals before definitive therapy when prolonged anesthesia is contraindicated. Berent and colleagues[40] reported on the use of locking loop nephrostomy catheters in 16 cats (18 kidneys) and four dogs (four kidneys). All but two dogs had ureteral obstructions. Because of the mobility of the feline kidney, 15 of 18 catheters were placed via laparotomy and three were placed percutaneously with ultrasound guidance. All four dogs had catheters placed percutaneously. Complications occurred in 2 of 20 (10%) cases including subcutaneous leakage in one cat and premature removal of the tube at home in one dog. No animals died related to the nephrostomy tube. Improvement in creatinine concentration was noted in 16 of 17 (94%) animals that survived surgery. Hence, with appropriate placement and care, nephrostomy tubes seem to be a good option for temporary urine diversion pending definitive intervention.

Ureteral stents are commonly used in people to prevent or relieve ureteral obstruction.[41,42] Over the last 10 years, the use of ureteral stents in veterinary medicine has been increasing.[13,43] Indications include treatment of benign and malignant ureteral obstructions and prevention of obstruction following percutaneous nephrolithotomy, sclerotherapy, and ureteral surgery. Stents result in passive dilation of the ureter, which helps prevent reobstruction from ureteroliths or nephroliths.[44] Endoscopic or percutaneous placement is commonly performed in the dog, whereas surgical placement is typically recommended in cats (**Figs. 2** and **3**).[13]

In dogs, there have been limited studies. In the largest report, 48 dogs (62 ureters) had endoscopic stent placement for benign obstructive disease caused by stones (49 ureters), stones and stricture (seven), stricture alone (five), and stone with a purulent plug (one).[45] Intraoperative complications occurred in 2 of 62 ureters (3%) resulting in ureteral tear (one) and perforation (one). Forty-seven of 48 dogs (98%) survived to discharge. Long-term complications included recurrent infections (13% vs 56% pre-stent), tissue proliferation at the UVJ (6%), ureteritis (6%), stent migration (4%), stent encrustation (4%), hematuria (4%), and stent fracture (2%). Fifteen ureters (23%) required either stent exchange (10 ureters) or SUB placement (five ureters). In a smaller study, 13 dogs (14 ureters) had stents placed endoscopically (11) or with surgical assistance (three).[46] Intraoperative complications occurred in two dogs (15%). Twelve of 13 dogs survived to discharge (92%). Long-term complications included recurrent infections (58% vs 85% prestent), tissue proliferation at the UVJ (42%), stent encrustation (8%), and stent migration (8%).

Overall, ureteral stents in dogs are successful in more than 90% of cases for treatment of benign obstruction, which is similar to surgery.[36] In the previous surgical

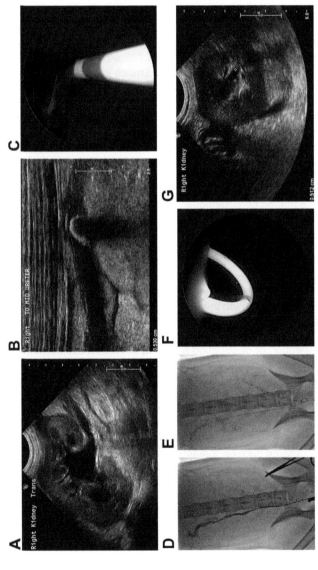

Fig. 2. Endoscopic stenting in a Dalmatian dog for ureteral obstruction secondary to a urate stone. Ultrasound shows moderate right hydronephrosis (*A*) and hydroureter with a stone present (*B*). Retroperitoneal effusion was also noted (not shown). (*C*) Under endoscopic and fluoroscopic guidance, a guidewire and ureteral catheter are inserted through the UVJ. (*D*) Retrograde pyeloureterogram reveals a proximal ureteral perforation likely causing the retroperitoneal effusion. A ureteral stent is placed (*E*) and urine drainage is noted during cystoscopy (*F*). (*G*) Transverse ultrasound the following day shows resolution of the right hydronephrosis.

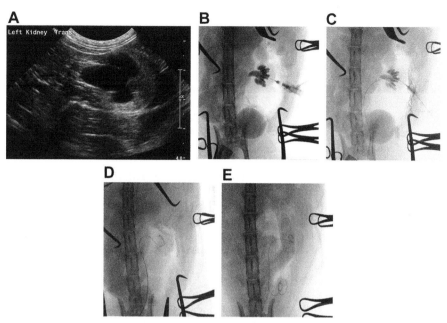

Fig. 3. Ureteral stenting in a cat for ureteral obstruction. (*A*) Ultrasound shows marked left hydronephrosis. (*B*) An intraoperative pyeloureterogram shows proximal ureteral obstruction. (*C*) A guidewire is passed antegrade from the kidney to the bladder and retrieved via cystotomy. (*D*) After antegrade passage of a dilator, the guidewire is reversed and coiled in the renal pelvis. (*E*) A 2.5F catheter ureteral stent is placed retrograde over the wire with the proximal coil in the renal pelvis and the distal stent coiled in the bladder.

study, 43% of dogs had postoperative infections (vs 54% presurgery), which is similar to the rates with stenting.[36] Given the minimally invasive nature of the procedure, stenting should be considered as an initial therapy for ureteral obstruction in dogs. Stents can typically be removed endoscopically if they are not needed long term or if complications occur. They are well tolerated in dogs with minimal lower urinary tract signs occurring.

Several variably sized studies have reported on outcomes of ureteral stenting in cats.[25,38,39,47–51] In the largest single study to date, ureteral stenting in 69 cats (79 ureters) with ureteral obstruction was reported.[49] Most cases were caused by ureterolithiasis (71%) with the remainder by stricture (13%), stone and stricture (15%), or purulent plug (1%). Stenting was successful in 95% of ureters, with four stents placed endoscopically. Thirty-five percent required an ureterotomy or neoureterocystostomy to facilitate placement. Six of 69 cats (8.7%) developed uroabdomen, of which two cats required an additional surgical procedure. Perioperative mortality was 7.5%. Long-term complications included reobstruction of ureters (19%), stent migration (6%), and dysuria (37%), which was temporary in all but one case. Stent exchange was required in 27% of ureters because of occlusion, migration, or irritation. In another large study, 43 cats had stents placed unilaterally (37) or bilaterally (six).[39] Nine cats had a concurrent ureterotomy and one had a neoureterocystostomy. Uroabdomen developed in 14% of cats and perioperative mortality was 9%. Long-term complications included dysuria (37%), chronic infections (26%), reobstruction (11%), and stent encrustation (5%). Seven of 43 cats (16%) required stent modification, replacement, or removal to relieve dysuria.

In a smaller study, Culp and colleagues[38] reported on 26 cats with unilateral (19) or bilateral (seven) stent placement. Ureterotomy was required in five cats (19%) to facilitate stent placement. Six cats developed abdominal effusion, with five having confirmed uroabdomen. Of the cats that developed a uroabdomen postoperative, four of those five had an ureterotomy performed. All six cats had an abdominal drain placed at the time of initial surgery and all effusions resolved spontaneously. Perioperative mortality rate was 7.6%. Long-term follow-up was not reported. In another study, Horowitz and colleagues[48] described ureteral stenting in 27 cats with six cats having bilateral stenting (33 ureters). Perioperative mortality was 11%. Long-term complication included dysuria (7%) and stent migration (4%). No cats developed reobstruction during the follow-up period.

Based on these studies, ureteral stenting in cats can be performed successfully with reduced perioperative mortality compared with ureteral surgery alone. The two larger studies each showed a high rate of dysuria (37%) and reobstruction (20%) with stenting, which was not seen in the study by Horowitz and colleagues,[48] although this included fewer cats. The dysuria often resolved with medical management including steroids, prazosin, analgesics, and/or amitriptyline. In some cases, stent removal or exchange may be needed. In addition, ureteral stenting in cats is technically challenging and sometimes requires ureterotomy or neoureterocystostomy to complete because of the small size of the normal feline ureter (0.4 mm).[52]

For these reasons, an SUB device was designed to improve management of ureteral obstructions in cats. The use of a subcutaneous ureteral bypass was first described in 1995 for human patients with ureteral obstructions secondary to urinary tract neoplasia as a means of avoidance of permanent nephrostomy tube placement.[53] The adapted veterinary device consists of a nephrostomy catheter placed in the renal pelvis or proximal ureter, a cystotomy catheter placed at the apex of the bladder, and a subcutaneous port that connects the system allowing percutaneous access for flushing and drainage (**Fig. 4**).

There are a small number of studies[26,48,54–56] or case reports[27,29,57,58] describing use of SUBs. In an initial study, SUBs were placed in 14 cats, with one having bilateral placement for ureteral obstruction.[48] Perioperative complications occurred in 6 of 14 (43%) including nephrostomy catheter leakage (two), nephropexy failure (one), nephrostomy catheter migration (one), and port leakage (one). Four of these five cats had revision surgery that corrected the leakage. The sixth cat developed obstruction of the SUB by a blood clot that was relieved using tissue plasminogen activator infusion. In the short term, dysuria was noted in 2 of 14 (14%) cats but resolved with medical management. No long-term complications were reported.

In a larger study reported in abstract form, 174 SUBs were placed in 137 cats with ureteral obstruction caused by ureteroliths (67%), strictures (13%), or both (20%).[55] Perioperative complications included device leakage (3.4%), catheter kinking (5%), and blood clot occlusion of the device (7.5%). Perioperative mortality was 6.3%. Long-term complications included catheter mineralization in 25%, with 13% requiring exchange because of reobstruction and dysuria in 8.2%.

Fages and colleagues[56] recently reported on ultrasound evaluation of the renal pelvis before and after SUB placement in 27 cats with 33 SUBs. Mean (range) pre-SUB pelvic size was 11.7 mm (0.9–41 mm). In the short- and long-term follow-up, the pelvic size was 2.4 mm (0–7.0 mm) and 1.7 (0–3.5 mm), respectively. In the follow-up period, nine cats (33.3%) had nonobstructive complications including hematuria (three) and urinary tract infection (three). Eight cats (29.6%) had an obstructive complication. In five cats, this was caused by kinking of the catheter, which necessitated surgical correction. The other three cats had partial

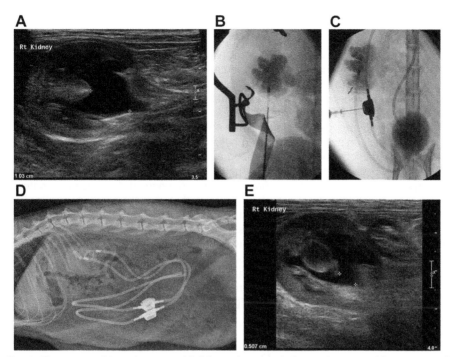

Fig. 4. Placement of SUBs in a cat with bilateral ureteral obstruction caused by congenital ureteropelvic junction stenosis. (*A*) Transverse ultrasound image of the right kidney shows severe hydronephrosis. (*B*) After an intraoperative pyeloureterogram, a locking-loop nephrostomy tube is placed through the caudal pole of the right kidney. (*C*) After placement of the cystostomy tube and connections to the subcutaneous port, the system is flushed under fluoroscopic imaging to check for leaks. (*D*) Postoperative radiograph after placement of bilateral SUBs. (*E*) Transverse ultrasound image of the right kidney 1 day after placement of SUBs shows marked improvement in hydronephrosis.

obstruction (two) and suspected renal carcinoma (one). Mean time to obstruction was 3.7 months.

In most of these studies, infection rates were not reported or difficult to discriminate from other treatments (eg, ureteral stenting). Anecdotally, a rate of 8% to 10% has been reported and cats with preoperative infections are more likely to have postoperative infections. Placement of a urethral catheter may increase the risk of infection. In a recent abstract of 19 cats with SUBs, 21% of cats developed an infection within 10 days of SUB placement, with 10% having chronic infections.[59] The incidence of infection is similar to that reported for ureteral stenting. Because SUBs are often easier to place than stents in cases with minimal ureteral dilation and are associated with less dysuria, it is recommended to place SUBs rather than stents in cats with ureteral obstructions.[13,48] Another potential advantage of SUBs is decreased surgical time.[54] Ultimately, the decision of surgery, stenting, or SUB placement should be evaluated on an individual basis after discussion of risks with the owner. Because most dogs are amenable to endoscopic or surgical ureteral stent placement, stenting is preferred. Given the higher rates of urinary tract infections in dogs, SUBs are typically reserved for cases that fail stenting or for palliation of advanced urinary tract neoplasia.

Obstructive Pyonephrosis

Pyonephrosis occurs when infection reaches the renal pelvis and there is subsequent ureteral obstruction resulting in renal pelvic abscessation. In dogs, obstruction is most often caused by uroliths, but may also be caused by strictures or cellular plugs.[46,60] Female dogs seem predisposed, likely associated with the increased risk of urinary tract infection. Pyonephrosis caused by ureterolith obstruction in four cats and stricture in one cat has been reported.[58,61] Animals may present with criteria of sepsis and cardiovascular derangements consistent with shock. Culture of urine obtained from the bladder may be negative for growth because of lack of drainage from the kidney or previous antibiotic therapy. Ultrasonographic findings were reported in 18 dogs with pyonephrosis compared with 10 dogs with hydronephrosis.[60] In pyonephrosis, findings included dispersed anechoic contents, dependent hyperechoic contents with a fluid-debris level, or hyperechoic contents that filled the renal pelvis (**Fig. 5**A). Conversely, all dogs with hydronephrosis had anechoic fluid.[60]

Drainage of the renal pelvis is necessary for pyonephrosis treatment, as with any other abscess. This is accomplished with nephrostomy tube placement, ureteral stenting, or SUB.[46,58,61] If a nephrostomy tube is placed, a second procedure is needed to relieve the ureteral obstruction. Ureteral stenting or SUB placement is beneficial in accomplishing both tasks. During stent placement, a ureteral catheter is passed into the renal pelvis for lavage (**Fig. 5**). If an SUB is placed, lavage is performed through the nephrostomy catheter.

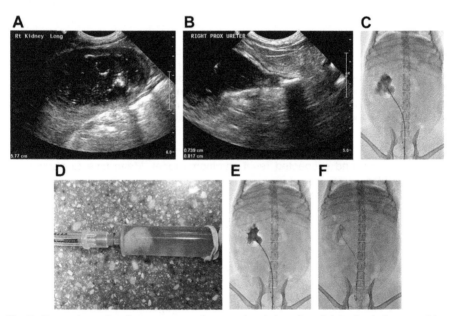

Fig. 5. Ureteral stenting for treatment of pyonephrosis in a dog. (*A*) Sagittal ultrasound image of the right kidney in a dog with severe hydronephrosis. Note the echogenic material in the dilated pelvis. (*B*) Ultrasound shows a stone causing obstruction in the proximal ureter. (*C*) A retrograde right pyeloureterogram is performed showing severe hydronephrosis with multiple filling defects. (*D*) Purulent material is aspirated from the right renal pelvis. (*E*) A pyeloureterogram is repeated after lavage of the right renal pelvis showing resolution of most of the filling defects. (*F*) A ureteral stent is placed to prevent reobstruction of the ureter.

In a recent report by Kuntz and colleagues,[46] 13 dogs with 14 obstructed ureters were treated for pyonephrosis with ureteral stenting. Endoscopic stent placement was successful in 11 of 12 (92%) dogs. In one dog, the guidewire could not pass the obstruction and the stent was placed surgically. One dog did not have endoscopic stenting attempted because of known septic peritonitis. All dogs survived to discharge. Seven of 12 dogs had recurrent infections, but all dogs were infection free on culture at last follow-up after appropriate antibiotic therapy. Stone analysis was performed in five dogs revealing calcium-based stones in three dogs, struvite-based in one dog, and mixed struvite and urate in one dog. In dogs with struvite stones, stents may be removed once the stones and infection have been resolved after appropriate antimicrobial and dissolution therapy. In dogs with other stones, the stent may need to remain in place to prevent reobstruction or to facilitate other minimally invasive stone treatment modalities, such as extracorporeal shockwave lithotripsy.

Malignant Ureteral Obstructions

Bladder tumors are uncommon in the dog and rare in the cat.[62] In the dog, transitional cell carcinoma is most common and frequently affects the trigone region. Most dogs die or are euthanized because of local progression and obstruction of the urinary tract rather than from metastatic disease.[62] Many cases are not considered surgical candidates, although radical cystectomy has been described.[63]

For dogs with ureteral obstruction, stenting of the affected ureter is performed. Because tumor typically obscures the UVJ, endoscopic placement is not performed in most cases. Instead, a percutaneous antegrade approach is used (**Fig. 6**). In 2011, Berent and colleagues[64] described placement of ureteral stents in 12 dogs (15 ureters) for malignant obstruction. In 11 of 12 dogs, stents were placed through a percutaneous antegrade approach. In one dog, the wire could not be manipulated out of the renal pelvis, requiring conversion to laparotomy. One dog required stent replacement secondary to stent migration. All dogs were discharged from the hospital. Median survival time from the date of diagnosis was 285 days (range, 10–1571 days) and from time of stent placement was 57 days (7–337 days). Dogs receiving chemotherapy before stenting had a longer median time from diagnosis to stent placement (180 days vs 3 days, respectively). No dogs died because of known stent complications or urinary obstruction.

Ectopic Ureters

EU are a congenital condition that results in malposition of the ureteral orifice caudal to the normal trigonal location. It is considered the most common cause of incontinence in juvenile dogs and cats.[65] Females are more commonly affected than males and usually diagnosed at a younger age. Males may be less likely to show incontinence because of increased pressure in the prostatic urethra and the longer length of urethra.

There are two anatomic EU variations: intramural and extramural. Intramural EU attach to the dorsal bladder wall at the trigone but then tunnel through the submucosa to open more distally in the bladder neck, urethra, or vestibule. Extramural EU bypass the trigone and attach directly to the urethra, vestibule, vagina, or uterus. Extramural EU are less common with reported incidence of 0% to 31% across multiple studies that did not include intramural EU only.[66–69] EU may be bilateral or unilateral with bilateral reported in a median of 51% (range, 32%–94%) of cases.[66–73]

Additional abnormalities including hydronephrosis, hydroureter, renal agenesis, renal dysplasia, and pelvic bladder may be present. Most cases in females (~90%) have a persistent paramesonephric remnant that may result in a vaginal septum or

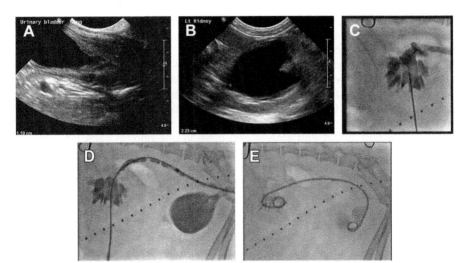

Fig. 6. Percutaneous ureteral stenting in a dog with obstruction from bladder transitional cell carcinoma. (*A*) Ultrasound of the bladder shows marked thickening in the trigone region. (*B*) Transverse ultrasound image of the left kidney shows marked hydronephrosis. (*C*) Using ultrasound and fluoroscopy, a percutaneous puncture of the renal pelvis for pyeloureterogram is performed followed by passage of a guidewire into the proximal ureter. (*D*) The guidewire is passed through the ureter into the bladder and out the urethra for through and through access. (*E*) The stent is placed in a retrograde direction.

a dual vagina (**Fig. 7**E).[73,74] Concurrent urinary tract infections have been reported at the time of diagnosis in a median of 65% of dogs (range, 38%–83%).[66,69,71–73,75] Of note, in a study of 16 male dogs with EU, only one (6%) had a urinary tract infection.

Diagnosis of EU relies on imaging of the urinary tract. Radiographic studies including excretory urography and retrograde vaginocystography were initially used but were only diagnostic in 60% to 70% of cases.[76] In a study by Lamb and Gregory,[76] ultrasound was comparable with contrast radiography for the detection of EU, but results were not confirmed by surgery. More recently, computed tomography excretory urography (CTEU) and cystoscopy have been shown to be superior for the diagnosis of EU.[65,77] For best results on CTEU, the animal should be positioned in sternal recumbency. A transurethral catheter is placed for removal of all urine and replacement with negative contrast (air) to better delineate the course of the ureters. Cystoscopy allows for better assessment of lower urinary tract abnormalities, such as persistent paramesonephric remnants, but does not allow evaluation of the upper urinary tract (**Fig. 7**).

Traditionally, surgical correction has been the treatment of EU with procedures including neoureterostomy, neoureterocystostomy, and ureteronephrectomy. Rates of full continence with surgery alone have ranged from 37% to 75% with higher rates typically reported in male dogs.[66–68,70,71,75] With the addition of medications, such as α-adrenergic agonists or estrogen supplements, continence rates range from 57% to 79%.[68,69,71] Postoperative complications are reported in 25% of dogs including uroabdomen.[68]

More recently, a cystoscopic-guided approach for treatment of EU has been described.[72,73,78] This approach is reserved for intramural EU only, which is typically determined by retrograde ureterography using fluoroscopy at the time of cystoscopic

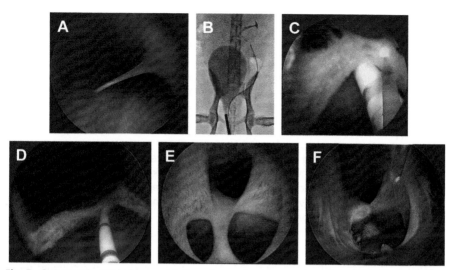

Fig. 7. Cystoscopic-guided laser ablation of an ectopic ureter in a dog. (*A*) Endoscopic view of the urethra showing an intramural ectopic ureter (lower right opening). (*B*) A contrast retrograde ureterogram and cystourethrogram confirm the intramural course of the ectopic ureter. (*C*) Under cystoscopic-guidance, a holmium:YAG laser is used to ablate the medial wall of the ectopic ureter using a ureteral catheter as a guide. (*D*) Cystoscopic image of the ureteral opening in the bladder after laser ablation of the ectopic ureter. (*E*) Endoscopic view of the vestibule shows a persistent paramesonephric remnant commonly seen in dogs with ectopic ureters and treated with laser ablation (*F*).

diagnosis of EU. Under cystoscopic-guidance, the medial wall of the EU is ablated using a laser (diode or holmium:YAG) until the ureteral orifice is positioned within the trigone of the bladder (see **Fig. 7**). During the procedure, persistent paramesonephric remnants can also be ablated, which may reduce the risk of incontinence and recurrent infections post-procedure (see **Fig. 7**E, F).[73,74] In male dogs this procedure may be done with flexible endoscopy but is challenging. A percutaneous perineal access technique has been described to allow rigid endoscopy for the ablation of the EU.[79] Potential complications include perforation of the urinary tract, UVJ stricture and hydronephrosis/hydroureter, or infections, although these are uncommon.

Use of cystoscopic-guided laser ablation (CLA) of EU was first described in four male dogs with incontinence.[78] Intramural EU were identified on CTEU in all dogs. All four dogs were continent immediately after the procedure. In a study by Smith and colleagues,[72] 16 female dogs underwent CLA for EU. Thirteen dogs had bilateral EU. Two dogs that received urethral collagen injection at the time of CLA and a third dog that subsequently had an ureteronephrectomy were excluded from outcome analysis. Four of 13 dogs (31%) were continent post-procedure. Five additional dogs were continent with the addition of phenylpropanolamine for a total continence rate of 69% (9 of 13).

Recently, a study evaluated CLA of intramural EU in 30 female dogs.[73] Eighteen of 30 dogs (60%) had bilateral EU. Complete continence was seen in 21 of 30 (70%) immediately after the procedure but decreased to 17 of 30 (57%) by 6 weeks. The addition of medications improved the rate to 17 of 30 (57%), transurethral bulking with collagen to 19 of 30 (63%), and placement of a urethral occluder device to 23 of 30 (77%). No major complications were noted.

Based on these studies, the outcome of CLA for EU is similar to surgery. There seem to be few complications and the procedure can often be performed on an outpatient basis. Post-procedure urethral edema and inflammation may result in initial continence in some dogs and subsequent recurrence as these resolve. The use of α-adrenergic agonists alone or combined with estrogen supplements may resolve incontinence in some dogs. In those that are still incontinent, injections of collagen or placement of a urethral occluder device should be considered.

SUMMARY

Interventional radiology and interventional endoscopy techniques have allowed the development of minimally invasive procedures to treat kidney and ureteral diseases in the dog and cat. In addition, the development of novel devices, such as the SUB, has increased the tools available. Early diagnosis and management of ureteral obstruction is important in preserving renal function.

REFERENCES

1. Stone EA, DeNovo RC, Rawlings CA. Massive hematuria of nontraumatic renal origin in dogs. J Am Vet Med Assoc 1983;183(8):868–71.
2. Hitt ME, Straw RC, Lattimer JC, et al. Idiopathic hematuria of unilateral renal origin in a dog. J Am Vet Med Assoc 1985;187(12):1371–3.
3. Holt PE, Lucke VM, Pearson H. Idiopathic renal haemorrhage in the dog. J Small Anim Pract 1987;28(4):253–63.
4. Mishina M, Watanabe T, Yugeta N, et al. Idiopathic renal hematuria in a dog; the usefulness of a method of partial occlusion of the renal artery. J Vet Med Sci 1997; 59(4):293–8.
5. Jennings PB, Mathey WS, Okerberg CV, et al. Idiopathic renal hematuria in a military working dog. Mil Med 1992;157(10):561–4.
6. Hawthorne J, deHaan J, Goring R, et al. Recurrent urethral obstruction secondary to idiopathic renal hematuria in a puppy. J Am Anim Hosp Assoc 1998;34(6): 511–4.
7. Berent AC, Weisse CW, Branter E, et al. Endoscopic-guided sclerotherapy for renal-sparing treatment of idiopathic renal hematuria in dogs: 6 cases (2010–2012). J Am Vet Med Assoc 2013;242(11):1556–63.
8. Di Cicco MF, Fetzer T, Secoura PL, et al. Management of bilateral idiopathic renal hematuria in a dog with silver nitrate. Can Vet J 2013;54(8):761–4.
9. Adelman LB, Bartges J, Whittemore JC. Povidone iodine sclerotherapy for treatment of idiopathic renal hematuria in two dogs. J Am Vet Med Assoc 2017;250(2): 205–10.
10. Heilmann RM, Thieman-Mankin KM, Cook AK. Bilateral renal sclerotherapy as a treatment option in a mixed breed male dog with idiopathic renal haematuria. Tierarztl Prax Ausg K Kleintiere Heimtiere 2015;43(4):253–9.
11. Berent A. New techniques on the horizon: Interventional radiology and interventional endoscopy of the urinary tract ('endourology'). J Feline Med Surg 2014; 16(1):51–65.
12. Araki M, Uehara S, Sasaki K, et al. Ureteroscopic management of chronic unilateral hematuria: a single-center experience over 22 years. PLoS One 2012;7(6): e36729.
13. Berent AC. Interventional radiology of the urinary tract. Vet Clin North Am Small Anim Pract 2016;46(3):567–96.

14. Berent A. Interventional treatment of idiopathic renal hematuria. In: Weisse C, Berent A, editors. Veterinary image-guided interventions. Oxford (England): Wiley Blackwell; 2015. p. 301–8.

15. Kyles AE, Hardie EM, Wooden BG, et al. Management and outcome of cats with ureteral calculi: 153 cases (1984–2002). J Am Vet Med Assoc 2005;226(6): 937–44.

16. Kyles AE, Hardie EM, Wooden BG, et al. Clinical, clinicopathologic, radiographic, and ultrasonographic abnormalities in cats with ureteral calculi: 163 cases (1984–2002). J Am Vet Med Assoc 2005;226(6):932–6.

17. Wen JG, Frøkiaer J, Jørgensen TM, et al. Obstructive nephropathy: an update of the experimental research. Urol Res 1999;27(1):29–39.

18. Kerr WS. Effect of complete ureteral obstruction for one week on kidney function. J Appl Physiol 1954;6(12):762–72.

19. Kerr WS. Effects of complete ureteral obstruction in dogs on kidney function. Am J Physiol 1956;184(3):521–6.

20. Vaughan ED, Gillenwater JY. Recovery following complete chronic unilateral ureteral occlusion: functional, radiographic and pathologic alterations. J Urol 1971; 106(1):27–35.

21. Miller JB, Marion DN, Gillenwater JY. Patterns of recovery of renal function after surgical relief of chronic bilateral partial ureteral obstruction. Invest Urol 1979; 17(1):69–74.

22. Fink RLW, Caridis DT, Chmiel R, et al. Renal impairment and its reversibility following variable periods of complete ureteric obstruction. Aust N Z J Surg 1980;50(1):77–83.

23. Leahy AL, Ryan PC, Mcentee GM, et al. Renal injury and recovery in partial ureteric obstruction. J Urol 1989;142(1):199–203.

24. Westropp JL, Ruby AL, Bailiff NL, et al. Dried solidified blood calculi in the urinary tract of cats. J Vet Intern Med 2006;20(4):828–34.

25. Zaid MS, Berent AC, Weisse C, et al. Feline ureteral strictures: 10 cases (2007–2009). J Vet Intern Med 2011;25(2):222–9.

26. Steinhaus J, Berent AC, Weisse C, et al. Clinical presentation and outcome of cats with circumcaval ureters associated with a ureteral obstruction. J Vet Intern Med 2015;29(1):63–70.

27. Kulendra E, Kulendra N, Halfacree Z. Management of bilateral ureteral trauma using ureteral stents and subsequent subcutaneous ureteral bypass devices in a cat. J Feline Med Surg 2014;16(6):536–40.

28. Lee N, Choi M, Keh S, et al. Bilateral congenital ureteral strictures in a young cat. Can Vet J 2014;55(9):841–4.

29. Johnson CM, Culp WTN, Palm CA, et al. Subcutaneous ureteral bypass device for treatment of iatrogenic ureteral ligation in a kitten. J Am Vet Med Assoc 2015;247(8):924–31.

30. Low WW, Uhl JM, Kass PH, et al. Evaluation of trends in urolith composition and characteristics of dogs with urolithiasis: 25,499 cases (1985–2006). J Am Vet Med Assoc 2010;236(2):193–200.

31. Adin CA, Herrgesell EJ, Nyland TG, et al. Antegrade pyelography for suspected ureteral obstruction in cats: 11 cases (1995–2001). J Am Vet Med Assoc 2003; 222(11):1576–81.

32. D'Anjou M-A, Bédard A, Dunn ME. Clinical significance of renal pelvic dilatation on ultrasound in dogs and cats. Vet Radiol Ultrasound 2011;52(1):88–94.

33. Anne-Archard N, Dunn M, d'Anjou M. Sonographic features of ureteral obstruction in cats. Cabo San Lucas (Mexico): Abstract VIRIES; 2017.

34. Quimby JM, Dowers K, Herndon AK, et al. Renal pelvic and ureteral ultrasono-graphic characteristics of cats with chronic kidney disease in comparison with normal cats, and cats with pyelonephritis or ureteral obstruction. J Feline Med Surg 2017;19(8):784–90.

35. Habling A, Byron JK. Imaging of the urinary tract. In: Weisse C, Berent A, editors. Veterinary image-guided interventions. Oxford (England): Wiley Blackwell; 2015. p. 263–88.

36. Snyder DM, Steffey MA, Mehler SJ, et al. Diagnosis and surgical management of ureteral calculi in dogs: 16 cases (1990–2003). N Z Vet J 2005;53(1):19–25.

37. Roberts SF, Aronson LR, Brown DC. Postoperative mortality in cats after uretero-lithotomy. Vet Surg 2011;40(4):438–43.

38. Culp WTN, Palm CA, Hsueh C, et al. Outcome in cats with benign ureteral ob-structions treated by means of ureteral stenting versus ureterotomy. J Am Vet Med Assoc 2016;249(11):1292–300.

39. Wormser C, Clarke DL, Aronson LR. Outcomes of ureteral surgery and ureteral stenting in cats: 117 cases (2006–2014). J Am Vet Med Assoc 2016;248(5): 518–25.

40. Berent AC, Weisse CW, Todd KL, et al. Use of locking-loop pigtail nephrostomy catheters in dogs and cats: 20 cases (2004–2009). J Am Vet Med Assoc 2012; 241(3):348–57.

41. Auge BK, Preminger GM. Ureteral stents and their use in endourology. Curr Opin Urol 2002;12(3):217–22.

42. Lam JS, Gupta M. Update on ureteral stents. Urology 2004;64(1):9–15.

43. Berent AC. Ureteral obstructions in dogs and cats: a review of traditional and new interventional diagnostic and therapeutic options. J Vet Emerg Crit Care (San An-tonio) 2011;21(2):86–103.

44. Vachon C, Defarges A, Brisson B, et al. Passive ureteral dilation and uretero-scopy after ureteral stent placement in five healthy Beagles. Am J Vet Res 2017;78(3):381–92.

45. Pavia P, Berent A, Weisse C, et al. Outcome following ureteral stenting in dogs with benign ureteral obstruction: 48 cases. San Diego (CA): Abstract ACVS; 2014.

46. Kuntz JA, Berent AC, Weisse CW, et al. Double pigtail ureteral stenting and renal pelvic lavage for renal-sparing treatment of obstructive pyonephrosis in dogs: 13 cases (2008–2012). J Am Vet Med Assoc 2015;246(2):216–25.

47. Nicoli S, Morello E, Martano M, et al. Double-J ureteral stenting in nine cats with ureteral obstruction. Vet J 2012;194(1):60–5.

48. Horowitz C, Berent A, Weisse C, et al. Predictors of outcome for cats with ureteral obstructions after interventional management using ureteral stents or a subcu-taneous ureteral bypass device. J Feline Med Surg 2013;15(12):1052–62.

49. Berent AC, Weisse CW, Todd K, et al. Technical and clinical outcomes of ureteral stenting in cats with benign ureteral obstruction: 69 cases (2006–2010). J Am Vet Med Assoc 2014;244(5):559–76.

50. Kulendra NJ, Syme H, Benigni L, et al. Feline double pigtail ureteric stents for management of ureteric obstruction: short- and long-term follow-up of 26 cats. J Feline Med Surg 2014;16(12):985–91.

51. Manassero M, Decambron A, Viateau V, et al. Indwelling double pigtail ureteral stent combined or not with surgery for feline ureterolithiasis: complications and outcome in 15 cases. J Feline Med Surg 2014;16(8):623–30.

52. Kochin EJ, Gregory CR, Wisner E, et al. Evaluation of a method of ureteroneocys-tostomy in cats. J Am Vet Med Assoc 1993;202(2):257–60.

53. Desgrandchamps F, Cussenot O, Meria P, et al. Subcutaneous urinary diversions for palliative treatment of pelvic malignancies. J Urol 1995;154(2):367–70.
54. Livet V, Pillard P, Goy-Thollot I, et al. Placement of subcutaneous ureteral by-passes without fluoroscopic guidance in cats with ureteral obstruction: 19 cases (2014–2016). J Feline Med Surg 2017;19(10):1030–9.
55. Berent A, Weisse C, Bagley D, et al. Subcutaneous ureteral bypass device (SUB) placement for benign ureteral obstruction in cats: 137 cats (174 obstructed ureters) (2009-2015). Jackson Hole (WY): Abstract VIRIES; 2016.
56. Fages J, Dunn M, Specchi S, et al. Ultrasound evaluation of the renal pelvis in cats with ureteral obstruction treated with a subcutaneous ureteral bypass: a retrospective study of 27 cases (2010–2015). J Feline Med Surg 2017. 1098612X17732900.
57. Heilmann RM, Pashmakova M, Lamb JH, et al. Subcutaneous ureteral bypass devices as a treatment option for bilateral ureteral obstruction in a cat with ureterolithiasis. Tierärztl Prax Kleintiere 2016;44(3):180–8.
58. Vedrine B. Perioperative occlusion of a subcutaneous ureteral bypass secondary to a severe pyonephrosis in a birman cat. Top Companion Anim Med 2017;32(2): 58–60.
59. Wolff EDS, Dorsch R, Knebel J, et al. Initial outcomes and complications of the subcutaneous ureteral bypass procedure at two university hospitals (2012–2015). Denver (CO): Abstract ACVIM; 2016.
60. Choi J, Jang J, Choi H, et al. Ultrasonographic features of pyonephrosis in dogs. Vet Radiol Ultrasound 2010;51(5):548–53.
61. Cray M, Berent AC, Weisse CW, et al. Treatment of pyonephrosis with a subcutaneous ureteral bypass device in four cats. J Am Vet Med Assoc 2018;252(6): 744–53.
62. Borrego JF. Urogenital and mammary gland tumors. Textbook of veterinary internal medicine. 8th edition. St. Louis (MO): Elsevier, Inc; 2017. p. 2119–26.
63. Ricardo Huppes R, Crivellenti LZ, Barboza De Nardi A, et al. Radical cystectomy and cutaneous ureterostomy in 4 dogs with trigonal transitional cell carcinoma: description of technique and case series. Vet Surg 2017;46(1):111–9.
64. Berent AC, Weisse C, Beal MW, et al. Use of indwelling, double-pigtail stents for treatment of malignant ureteral obstruction in dogs: 12 cases (2006–2009). J Am Vet Med Assoc 2011;238(8):1017–25.
65. Cannizzo KL, McLoughlin MA, Mattoon JS, et al. Evaluation of transurethral cystoscopy and excretory urography for diagnosis of ectopic ureters in female dogs: 25 cases (1992–2000). J Am Vet Med Assoc 2003;223(4):475–81.
66. Ho LK, Troy GC, Waldron DR. Clinical outcomes of surgically managed ectopic ureters in 33 dogs. J Am Anim Hosp Assoc 2011;47(3):196–202.
67. Anders KJ, McLoughlin MA, Samii VF, et al. Ectopic ureters in male dogs: review of 16 clinical cases (1999–2007). J Am Anim Hosp Assoc 2012;48(6):390–8.
68. Reichler IM, Eckrich Specker C, Hubler M, et al. Ectopic ureters in dogs: clinical features, surgical techniques and outcome. Vet Surg 2012;41(4):515–22.
69. Noël SM, Claeys S, Hamaide AJ. Surgical management of ectopic ureters in dogs: clinical outcome and prognostic factors for long-term continence*. Vet Surg 2017;46(5):631–41.
70. Holt PE, Moore AH. Canine ureteral ectopia: an analysis of 175 cases and comparison of surgical treatments. Vet Rec 1995;136(14):345–9.
71. Mayhew PD, Lee KCL, Gregory SP, et al. Comparison of two surgical techniques for management of intramural ureteral ectopia in dogs: 36 cases (1994–2004). J Am Vet Med Assoc 2006;229(3):389–93.

72. Smith AL, Radlinsky MG, Rawlings CA. Cystoscopic diagnosis and treatment of ectopic ureters in female dogs: 16 cases (2005–2008). J Am Vet Med Assoc 2010;237(2):191–5.

73. Berent AC, Weisse C, Mayhew PD, et al. Evaluation of cystoscopic-guided laser ablation of intramural ectopic ureters in female dogs. J Am Vet Med Assoc 2012; 240(6):716–25.

74. Burdick S, Berent AC, Weisse C, et al. Endoscopic-guided laser ablation of vestibulovaginal septal remnants in dogs: 36 cases (2007–2011). J Am Vet Med Assoc 2014;244(8):944–9.

75. Stone EA, Mason LK. Surgery of ectopic ureters: types, method of correction, and postoperative results. J Am Anim Hosp Assoc 1990;26(1):81–8.

76. Lamb CR, Gregory SP. Ultrasonographic findings in 14 dogs with ectopic ureter. Vet Radiol Ultrasound 1998;39(3):218–23.

77. Samii VF, McLoughlin MA, Mattoon JS, et al. Digital fluoroscopic excretory urography, digital fluoroscopic urethrography, helical computed tomography, and cystoscopy in 24 dogs with suspected ureteral ectopia. J Vet Intern Med 2004; 18(3):271–81.

78. Berent AC, Mayhew PD, Porat-Mosenco Y. Use of cystoscopic-guided laser ablation for treatment of intramural ureteral ectopia in male dogs: four cases (2006–2007). J Am Vet Med Assoc 2008;232(7):1026–34.

79. Tong K, Weisse C, Berent AC. Rigid urethrocystoscopy via a percutaneous fluoroscopic-assisted perineal approach in male dogs: 19 cases (2005–2014). J Am Vet Med Assoc 2016;249(8):918–25.

Interventional Management of Urethral Obstructions

Matthew W. Beal, DVM

KEYWORDS

- Urethral stent • Urethral obstruction • Transitional cell carcinoma • Urethral stricture
- Incontinence • Malignant urethral obstruction • Benign urethral obstruction
- Interventional radiology

KEY POINTS

- Lower urinary tract obstruction can represent a life-threatening emergency. Patient stabilization through appropriate medical therapies for the management of hyperkalemia, metabolic acidosis, and uremia are critical before definitive intervention.
- Malignant urethral obstruction is the most common indication for urethral stent placement in dogs and cats.
- Urethral stent placement offers a minimally invasive, image-guided alternative to prolonged urinary diversion via a cystostomy tube in select patients.
- The most common complication of urethral stent placement is urinary incontinence.
- Percutaneous antegrade urethral access can help facilitate urethral access for catheterization or stent placement when retrograde access to the urethra and bladder is not possible.

INTRODUCTION

Lower urinary tract obstruction is a common cause of morbidity and mortality in small animal patients. Urolithiasis in dogs and obstructive feline lower urinary tract disease in cats are the most common causes of lower urinary tract obstruction, and these conditions can be managed through a combination of medical, dietary, and surgical intervention. Other conditions, including neoplasia and benign urethral strictures, may also cause urinary obstruction. These conditions create therapeutic challenges that, in the past, have necessitated long-term urinary diversion via a cystostomy tube or complex surgical interventions. Urethral stent placement offers therapeutic alternative to these traditional treatment methods.[1–8] Patient selection and screening is critical to optimizing outcomes. Stent placement is performed using image guidance, with fluoroscopy being preferred, although digital radiography is a described alternative.[8] Urethral stents are placed almost exclusively via a retrograde approach using the urethral orifice, but an antegrade access approach is also possible. The following paragraphs detail

Department of Small Animal Clinical Sciences, Michigan State University, 736 Wilson Road, East Lansing, MI 48824-1314, USA
E-mail address: bealmatt@cvm.msu.edu

Vet Clin Small Anim 48 (2018) 863–874
https://doi.org/10.1016/j.cvsm.2018.05.006
0195-5616/18/© 2018 Elsevier Inc. All rights reserved.

stabilization, patient selection, diagnostic workup, placement technique, expected outcomes, and complications for patients undergoing urethral stent placement.

STABILIZATION OF THE PATIENT WITH LOWER URINARY TRACT OBSTRUCTION

Lower urinary tract obstruction can be life-threatening due to hyperkalemia, metabolic acidosis, and uremia. Medical management of these conditions and stabilization of the patient is critical before definitive intervention. Irrespective of the cause of lower urinary tract obstruction, initial stabilization may include the following:

- Volume expansion with balanced isotonic crystalloid solutions or 0.9% saline to restore intravascular volume, treat dehydration, and rapidly dilute the elevated concentration of potassium in the blood.
- Calcium gluconate (20–60 mg/kg intravenously [IV] over 1–3 minutes) works very rapidly to protect the heart from the effects of hyperkalemia.
- Regular insulin (0.25 u/kg IV) and dextrose (0.25–0.5 g/kg IV) will help to redistribute potassium intracellularly and has a more delayed effect than volume expansion and calcium gluconate administration (onset time approximately 20 minutes).
- Sodium bicarbonate (0.1 × Body Weight (kg) × Base Deficit) given over 30 minutes will also help redistribute potassium intracellularly while also managing severe metabolic acidosis. The author will use bicarbonate if the pH is less than 7.1 or there are clinical manifestations of severe metabolic acidosis. Onset time is similar to insulin/dextrose.
- Urinary diversion via a urinary catheter or cystostomy tube has a very slow effect on lowering serum potassium concentration and is generally delayed until hemodynamic stability has been achieved. If possible, the use of an end-hole catheter, or cutting off the closed end of a red rubber or Foley catheter, will make subsequent wire access for urethral stent placement easier.

INDICATIONS AND PATIENT SELECTION FOR URETHRAL STENT PLACEMENT

Fortunately, dogs and cats with neoplastic urethral obstruction and urethral stricture often have gradual and progressive signs of lower urinary tract obstruction such that clients usually recognize signs of lower urinary tract disease before complete obstruction occurs. Once stabilization has been performed, the cause of the urethral obstruction must be determined. A comprehensive discussion of the causes and diagnostic techniques used for workup of dogs and cats presenting with urethral obstruction is beyond the scope of this article. In general, a combination of historical findings; physical examination findings, including a rectal examination to evaluate the pelvic urethra and a vaginal examination in females; radiographic; ultrasonographic; urethrocystoscopic (with biopsy); and positive contrast urethrocystographic imaging allow for the determination of the underlying cause of the lower urinary tract obstruction.

Urethral stents may be placed for the following conditions:

- Urethral obstruction due to transitional cell carcinoma, prostatic carcinoma, leiomyoma, or other neoplastic conditions of the urethra.
- External urethral compression secondary to metastatic intrapelvic lymphadenopathy.
- Benign urethral obstruction associated with previous urethral trauma (including iatrogenic), previous surgery, reflex dyssynergia, and proliferative urethritis.

Of critical importance before stent placement is the conclusive determination that the patient is indeed obstructed. Animals with lower urinary tract neoplasia often have stranguria and pollakiuria due to local inflammation and the presence of the mass. These signs are identical to those that are truly obstructed. However, many may simply have lower urinary tract signs and may not actually be obstructed. Only about 10% of dogs with lower urinary tract neoplasia develop urinary obstruction. Sometimes, obstruction is obvious and the bladder is large, firm, and/or painful and the owner notes decreased urine production. Other times, only lower urinary tract signs predominate. In these cases, the author finds it helpful to evaluate the bladder with ultrasound both before and after multiple attempts to void. Failure to empty the bladder despite multiple attempts indicates, at minimum, a partial obstruction, and stent placement should be considered. Dogs with a very poor urine stream that still empty likely have a partial obstruction and urethral stent placement should be considered.

Of note, in cases of partial obstruction, some oncologists prefer to treat with medical (nonsteroidal antiinflammatory drugs) or radiation therapy in an attempt to decrease tumor size and palliate the signs of obstruction and dysuria while urine is diverted via a urinary catheter. The success rate of these methods is currently unknown.

Workup of the patient with suspected partial or complete urinary obstruction should be guided by the presumed diagnosis but should, at minimum, include complete blood count, serum biochemical profile, urinalysis, and urine culture. Radiographic or computed tomographic assessment of the chest and abdomen should be strongly considered to assess for metastatic disease. In patients with suspected neoplasia, ultrasonographic assessment of the bladder and upper urinary tract is critical to rule out concurrent ureteral obstruction. Dogs with concurrent ureteral and urethral obstruction will require an upper urinary tract intervention (stent, neoureterocystostomy, or subcutaneous ureteral bypass) concurrent with urethral stent placement.

URETHRAL STENT PLACEMENT TECHNIQUE

1. Urethral stent placement is optimally performed with the aid of fluoroscopic guidance. A technique for digital radiographic stent placement has been described; however, the lack of immediate feedback and the lack of ability to acquire a series of images throughout urethrocystography makes this technique challenging.[8] Urethral stent placement can be performed in female cats using the same techniques as described for dogs. Male cats that have not had a prior perineal urethrostomy may require normograde access to the urethra via the bladder due to the small urethral size, which is less than the size of the self-expanding stent delivery system. However, stent deployment using a balloon-expandable metallic stent placed retrograde has been described in cats (**Figs. 1–4**).[5,6]
2. The patient should be placed under general anesthesia and monitored routinely. Patients undergoing stent placement should be stabilized medically as described earlier. Appropriate measures should be undertaken to prevent hypothermia through convective and conductive means while not interfering with image guidance. Perioperative antibiotics should be used.
3. Appropriately clip the caudal abdomen free of hair in both male and female dogs. If retrograde access is not possible, which is uncommon, antegrade urethral catheterization may be performed (described later). In the male, the prepuce should be completely clipped and lavaged and prepared with a margin free of hair comparable to what is needed for abdominal surgery. A wide 4- to 6-inch field around the vulva should be surgically prepared in the female. If a urinary catheter remains in place, it should be aseptically prepared to be in the operative field.
4. The patient is positioned in either right or left lateral recumbency depending on the layout of the imaging suite where the procedure is being performed. A 5Fr marker

A   B

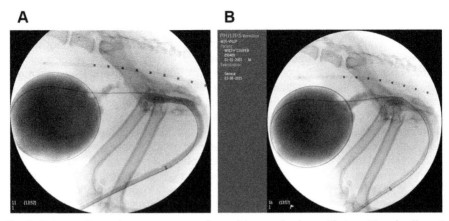

Fig. 1. Retrograde urethrocystogram performed in a male dog with transitional cell carcinoma. Note the presence of the marker catheter in the colon, the hydrophilic guidewire across the obstruction, and the vascular sheath in the distal urethra. Note that the bladder is well distended to delineate the trigone from urethra. The filling defect extends into the bladder (*A*). The urethral stent was placed from bladder and spanned to the unobstructed portion of urethra (*B*).

catheter can be placed inside a well-lubricated 12Fr red-rubber catheter and advanced into the rectum and up the descending colon using digital and fluoroscopic guidance. Optimal positioning is confirmed fluoroscopically and will include the radiopaque markings being positioned at a level from mid-bladder through the pelvic urethra. The marker catheter (positioned at the same level as the urethra and bladder) is used to calibrate the measurement software included in the imaging hardware. A tampon should be placed in the rectum to help prevent fecal material entering the draped area in female dogs. A final surgical preparation should be performed.

5. The operators should gown and glove and wear a cap and mask as is routine for a surgical procedure.

6. Draping in the male dog should include 4″ on all sides of the prepuce. The penis will need to be extruded, necessitating access to the prepuce. If percutaneous antegrade urethral catheterization is necessary, this method for draping will allow for appropriate access. In the female dog, draping is performed to create a sterile field including the ventral abdomen extending from the umbilicus to the pelvic inlet to prepare for antegrade urethral access if necessary. A sterile field should also be created surrounding the vulva. When using long wires and catheters necessary for this procedure, a large area of the table cranial to the penis or caudal to the vulva will be needed to ensure that the catheters and wires remain sterile. The image intensifier/flat panel detector should be covered with a sterile dome cover.

7. If the patient has an indwelling urinary catheter with an open end, a 0.035″ angled tip, standard stiffness, hydrophilic guidewire (HGW) may be advanced up the catheter and into the bladder. The catheter is then removed over the HGW. If the patient does not have a urinary catheter in place, the HGW may be advanced up the urethra in the male and coiled in the bladder. In the female dog, the author finds it easiest to catheterize the distal urethra digitally with an end-hole catheter appropriate for the size of the patient and then to feed the HGW up that catheter and the remainder of the way into the urethra and subsequently, the bladder. The catheter can then be discarded. Depending on the location of the obstruction and

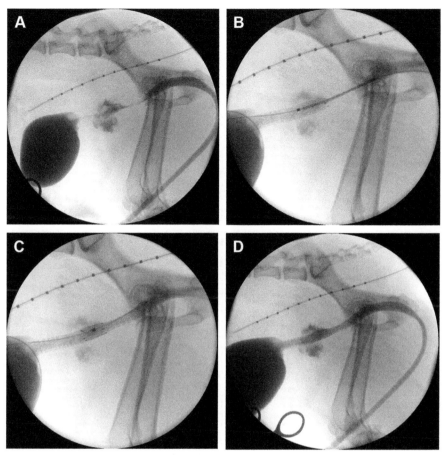

Fig. 2. Lateral fluoroscopic images of a large breed male dog demonstrating the length of obstruction (*A*) and need for 2 urethral stents to be placed to span the obstruction. Note that the first stent has been deployed and without loss of wire access, the second is placed caudal to the first stent with approximately 1 cm of overlap (*B*). On completion of deployment of the second stent (*C*), patency of the urethra is confirmed with a retrograde cystourethrogram (*D*).

the severity of the obstruction, fluoroscopic guidance and manual direction of the guidewire may be necessary. Use of a torque device placed on the HGW will facilitate manipulation and guidance of the wire into the bladder. Urethrocystoscopy may also be used to facilitate wire access to the bladder if needed. Next, a 4 to 10 cm 6 to 8F vascular sheath and dilator should be advanced over the HGW and into the urethra (male) or bladder (female). The dilator is removed and, in the male, the sheath is secured to the prepuce with suture. The vascular sheath will serve as a port for repeated reintroduction of different devices necessary for the procedure and will also partially occlude the urethra. In the female dog, in addition to these functions, the vascular sheath is also used to perform urethrography via the side-arm of the sheath.

8. Percutaneous antegrade urethral access (PAUC) may be required if retrograde access is not possible. Please see later discussion for a description of this technique.

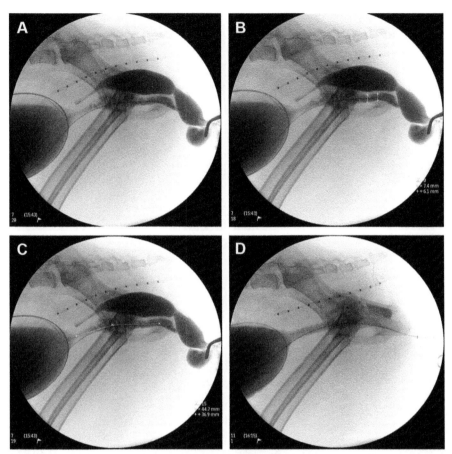

Fig. 3. Retrograde cystourethrogram from a female dog demonstrating obstruction spanning most of the urethral length, which was confirmed with cystoscopy (*A*). Measurements of normal urethral diameter (*B*) and length of obstruction (*C*) were used to determine stent size, which was an 8 mm × 80 mm laser cut urethral stent (*D*).

9. Bladder distention and cystourethrography:
   a. In the male dog, a 4 to 5Fr Berenstein catheter is advanced over the HGW and through the vascular sheath. The HGW is removed and the bladder is distended to a large diameter with iodinated contrast medium in saline. The contrast agent should be diluted enough that the guidewire should be visible within the bladder. The importance of this step of the procedure cannot be overemphasized. Failure to distend the bladder will result in an inability to discern the trigone from the proximal urethra and will result in malpositioning of the stent within the bladder. Then, while firmly compressing the penis around the vascular sheath and forcefully injecting a 1:1 mixture of iodinated contrast medium and saline through the Berenstein catheter, the catheter is withdrawn back into the vascular sheath. The entire urethra should be imaged. This procedure is recorded fluoroscopically. The goal of this phase of the procedure is to achieve maximum dilation of the urethra such that the maximum diameter of the healthy urethra adjacent to the area of obstruction can be determined and so that the length of the obstruction can be measured.

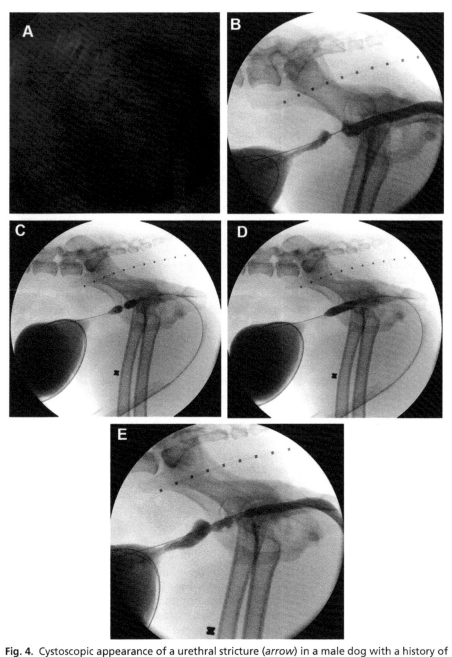

Fig. 4. Cystoscopic appearance of a urethral stricture (*arrow*) in a male dog with a history of pelvic trauma (*A*), through which only a 0.035″ hydrophilic guidewire could be placed. Retrograde urethrocystography confirming the length and severity of the obstruction (*B*). Balloon dilation of the urethral stricture over an HGW, showing an initial waist (*C*), then complete opening of the balloon (*D*). Repeat retrograde urethrocystography demonstrating restoration of luminal patency, (*E*) although irregularity in the mucosa persists.

b. In the female dog, the vascular sheath and dilator will usually extend into the bladder neck or bladder when advanced over the HGW. To perform cystourethrography, the dilator is removed and the side-arm of the vascular sheath is forcefully injected as the sheath is withdrawn over the HGW to maximally distend the short female urethra. The HGW remains in place to maintain bladder access. If the sheath needs to be reintroduced into the urethra, it should be done over the HGW with the dilator in place.

10. Measurements: the location of the obstruction should be identified and its location noted in relation to anatomic landmarks (vertebral bodies, pelvic landmarks, etc) or a radiopaque stent guide placed on the table ventral and parallel to the bladder and urethra. Measurements of the length of the obstruction and the diameter of the normal urethra both cranial and caudal to the obstruction should be ascertained. Often, the cranial aspect of the obstruction is in the bladder. In this scenario, the caudal normal urethra diameter is used to determine stent diameter. The length of the obstruction should also be measured. It is critically important to use the standard measurements on the marker catheter in the colon to calibrate measurement software built into the imaging system. Failure to perform this step is a common source of error in determining appropriate urethral stent size.

11. Stent selection:

a. Malignant urethral obstruction: laser-cut, self-expanding metallic (nitinol) stents (SEMS) are most commonly used for relieving malignant urethral obstructions. These stents do not foreshorten on deployment, meaning that their length on the delivery system will be the same as their deployed length. Normal urethral diameter adjacent to the obstruction is used to determine stent diameter. Stent diameter should be chosen to exceed the adjacent urethral dimension by 0% to 20%. The length of the stent is chosen to exceed the length of the obstruction by approximately 1 cm on either side of it.

b. Benign urethral obstruction: dogs with benign urethral obstruction have been historically treated with both balloon dilation and urethral stent placement.[2,7] Dogs with urethral stricture treated by balloon dilation may require multiple treatments and the procedure is not uniformly successful. Because of this, SEMS placement has been described as an alternative. SEMS are generally recommended for urethral stricture (over balloon-expandable metallic stents); however, tissue ingrowth may occur in some patients resulting in recurrent obstruction and use of a covered SEMS (CSEMS) will prevent this. Retrievable CSEMS are also available. Other causes of benign obstruction including suspected reflex dyssynergia and proliferative urethritis have also been treated with SEMS placement.

12. Stent deployment: the stent should be prepared by lubricating the external surface with saline and flushing all ports with saline. This will help ensure that it advances over the HGW, through the sheath, and into position. The stent is advanced over the HGW and centered on the area of known obstruction using the anatomic landmarks or stent guide as noted in (10) earlier. It is important to remember that laser cut urethral stents are not reconstrainable, meaning they cannot be recaptured or repositioned once deployment has been initiated. The stent is deployed by simply withdrawing the outer sheath that covers the stent (attached to the "Y" piece of the stent) allowing it to expand. It is critically important that the operator does not push the stent out of the delivery system. Often, the cranial aspect of the obstruction is in the bladder neck, in which case the cranial most aspect of the stent should be advanced just into the bladder and deployed until it achieves a conical appearance (about ½–1 cm). Back tension is

then applied to the delivery system to pull the stent back into the area of obstruction. While maintaining light back tension, the remainder of the stent is deployed across the obstruction. Back tension is critical to prevent the stent from being deployed into the bladder. The delivery system can be withdrawn over the HGW using fluoroscopic guidance.

13. Challenges: rarely, the mass extends the entire length of the urethra. This tends to occur in female dogs. When this occurs, the only options are to stent the entire urethra, raising concerns for incontinence or to stent approximately 2/3 to 3/4 of the urethra (partial obstruction length stenting), being sure to include the portion of the urethra that seems most severely obstructed. Most often, the most severe portion of the obstruction is proximal; however, urethrography and urethroscopy can help make this determination. Should the option for partial obstruction length stenting be chosen, the patient should be recovered from anesthesia to assess the efficacy of stent placement. If the stent does not clinically relieve the obstruction using this technique, a second stent can be placed to extend the remaining length of the urethra. If a client can only consider a single procedure, the entire urethra may be spanned by the stent. If the obstruction extends into the vagina, the stent will need to be deployed to extend to the caudal most aspect of the obstruction. The author generally avoids deploying the stent 1 cm beyond the obstruction due to discomfort that may accompany stent deployment into the vagina.

14. Postprocedure urethrocystography: retrograde urethrocystography may be performed via the vascular sheath positioned in the distal urethra in both male and female dogs. This study may be performed in both lateral and ventrodorsal recumbency. Contrast should flow unobstructed into the bladder. Once confirmed, all devices should be removed from the urinary system. This procedure is followed by applying gentle pressure to the bladder to visualize unobstructed expression of urine. Both studies should be documented in the medical record.

15. Devices such as urinary catheters should be avoided after stent placement to avoid trauma to the stent or entanglement of the stent and urinary catheter. If necessary for any reason (rare), fluoroscopic guidance should be considered during urinary catheterization and avoiding use of a Foley catheter should be very strongly considered.

16. Most dogs undergoing urethral stent placement are monitored until it is confirmed that they are effectively emptying their bladder and the degree of urinary continence can be assessed. This may be accomplished either on an outpatient or on an inpatient basis. Pain medication after this procedure is generally not necessary.

EXPECTED OUTCOME AND COMPLICATIONS

Although the minimally invasive nature of urethral stenting is attractive, the financial investment in urethral stent placement can be significant. In cases of malignant urethral obstruction, clients must recognize that the stent merely relieves the obstruction and palliates the patient and that it does not treat the tumor specifically. In relieving the obstruction, however, the period of good quality of life is prolonged.

Most animals will be continent after urethral stent placement. Even still, incontinence is a significant risk after urethral stent placement, which can range from mild to severe. Estimates of incontinence rates range from 25% to 64%.[3,7] Clients must accept the real risk of incontinence before stent placement because laser cut urethral stents cannot be removed once placed. For clients that cannot accept this risk, the author strongly advocates for an alternate means of sustained bladder decompression such as cystostomy tube placement. Some patients are incontinent before stent placement and can be expected to be incontinent after placement as well. If incontinence persists beyond 1 week, therapy with phenylpropanolamine or use of a bulking agent may be considered.[9] In animals that have had chronic obstruction and chronic bladder distention, bladder atony may be present. Once the obstruction is relieved, bethanechol may be administered to improve tone of the urinary bladder. Maintaining bladder decompression is an often-overlooked component of this medical strategy and may require the use of an indwelling urinary catheter while awaiting the return of bladder tone.

In dogs with malignant obstruction, clients should also be prepared for the possibility that some degree of the stranguria present preprocedure (from the local inflammation in the bladder) may persist after procedure. Intermittent hematuria may also occur due to the vascular nature of some masses.

Repeat obstruction of the urinary tract due to ingrowth of tumor through the interstices of the stent, overgrowth of tumor beyond the stent, or development of a new mass beyond the stent is very rare. The author estimates the incidence of this complication as less than 10%. Clients should be made aware of this unlikely possibility because the biological behavior of a given tumor is often difficult to determine.

Finally, in animals with masses that also involve the bladder, progression to involve ureteral obstruction may occur. Although uncommon, this problem would require additional intervention through neoureterocystostomy, subcutaneous ureteral bypass, or ureteral stent placement.

Expected survival after stent placement is difficult to predict for an individual patient and is best determined by the presence of the stage of the neoplasia (in those cases) and comorbid conditions. Chemotherapeutics and the use of nonsteroidal antiinflammatory medications are expected to prolong life in dogs with neoplastic obstruction. Animals with benign urethral obstruction are expected to survive independent of their underlying condition.[2,3]

Percutaneous Antegrade Urethral Access

PAUC is a useful technique for gaining access to the urethra when standard retrograde techniques are not possible.[10] Most often, the technique is used for difficult retrograde catheterization due to trigonal and urethral neoplasia and urethral disruption due to trauma or iatrogenic causes. The technique may also be used to gain access to the proximal urethra and trigone for stent placement in male cats where the standard delivery system may be too large to deliver the stent retrograde.

Percutaneous Antegrade Urethral Access Technique

1. The patient should be placed under general anesthesia to ensure adequate time and maintenance of sterile technique during this procedure.
2. The patient is positioned in lateral recumbency. The abdomen is prepared as if for exploratory laparotomy and draped such that the caudolateral abdomen is accessible. Long drapes should extend cranial and caudal to the patient to ensure that the HGW remains sterile during the procedure. A dome cover should be placed over the image intensifier/flat panel detector. The operators should wear cap, mask, and gowns/gloves to prevent contamination of the HGW or other devices introduced over it.
3. Using fluoroscopic guidance, a suitable puncture site on the ventral aspect of the apex to body of the bladder is identified. The proposed insertion site may be infused with lidocaine and a 3 to 4 mm incision is made in the skin. Blunt dissection with a hemostat will help decrease tissue drag should devices need to be advanced over the HGW.

4. The bladder is punctured using an 18 g 2″ IV catheter or an 18 g puncture needle at an angle such that the bevel is directed toward the trigone.
5. A small sample of urine should be aspirated from the bladder and, if needed, submitted for urinalysis and culture. Acquisition of urine also ensures that the needle/catheter has penetrated the lumen and is not merely submucosal.
6. Sterile, iodinated contrast media and 0.9% saline is infused such that the trigone is clearly visible and at a concentration such that the HGW remains clearly visible.
7. A 0.035″ × 150 cm angled, standard stiffness, HGW is advanced through the catheter or puncture needle and is directed toward the trigone. Use of a torque device will facilitate smooth control of the HGW. If using a puncture needle, caution must be exercised not to withdraw the HGW through the puncture needle because the hydrophilic coating may be sheared off, remaining in the bladder as a foreign body.
8. If needed, advancing a 4Fr 65 cm Berenstein catheter (angled) over the guidewire can provide additional directional capability and rigidity for negotiating difficult stenoses.
9. The HGW is advanced across the region of pathology and allowed to exit the urethral orifice.
10. If the goal of PAUC is retrograde catheterization, it is then performed over the HGW and the HGW is subsequently removed. If the goal of PAUC is to facilitate stent placement either antegrade or retrograde, the HGW should remain in place for the duration of the procedure. If PAUC fails, a cystostomy tube may be placed over the HGW to allow for urinary diversion until definitive therapy to resolve the underlying pathology can be performed.

REFERENCES

1. Weisse C, Berent A, Todd K, et al. Evaluation of palliative stenting for management of malignant urethral obstructions in dogs. J Am Vet Med Assoc 2006; 229:226–34.
2. Hill TL, Berent AC, Weisse CW. Evaluation of urethral stent placement for benign urethral obstructions in dogs. J Vet Intern Med 2014;28(5):1384–90.
3. Blackburn AL, Berent AC, Weisse CW, et al. Evaluation of outcome following urethral stent placement for the treatment of obstructive carcinoma of the urethra in dogs: 42 cases (2004-2008). J Am Vet Med Assoc 2013;242(1):59–68.
4. McMillan SK, Knapp DW, Ramos-Vara JA, et al. Outcome of urethral stent placement for management of urethral obstruction secondary to transitional cell carcinoma in dogs: 19 cases (2007-2010). J Am Vet Med Assoc 2012; 241(12):1627–32.
5. Brace MA, Weisse C, Berent A. Preliminary experience with stenting for management of non-urolith urethral obstruction in eight cats. Vet Surg 2014;43(2): 199–208.
6. Newman RG, Mehler SJ, Kitchell BE, et al. Use of a balloon-expandable metallic stent to relieve malignant urethral obstruction in a cat. J Am Vet Med Assoc 2009; 234(2):236–9.
7. Weisse C. Urethral stenting. In: Weisse C, Berent A, editors. Veterinary image guided interventions. Wiley Blackwell; 2015. p. 373–82.
8. Radhakrishnan A. Urethral stenting for obstructive uropathy utilizing digital radiography for guidance: feasibility and clinical outcome in 26 dogs. J Vet Intern Med 2017;31(2):427–33.

9. Kilpatrick S, Hill T. Submucosal collagen injection for management of urinary incontinence following urethral stent placement. Top Companion Anim Med 2017; 32(2):55–7.
10. Holmes ES, Weisse C, Berent AC. Use of fluoroscopically guided percutaneous antegrade urethral catheterization for the treatement of urethral obstruction in male cats: 9 cases (2000-2009). J Am Vet Med Assoc 2012;241:603–7.

FURTHER READINGS

Holmes ES. Percutaneous antegrade urethral catheterization. In: Weisse C, Berent A, editors. Veterinary image guided interventions. Wiley Blackwell; 2015. p. 419–22.

Minimally Invasive Management of Uroliths in Cats and Dogs

Andréanne Cléroux, DMV

KEYWORDS

- Urolith • Extracorporeal shockwave lithotripsy (ESWL)
- Endoscopic nephrolithotomy (ENL) • Basket retrieval • Laser lithotripsy
- Percutaneous cystolithotomy (PCCL) • Endourology

KEY POINTS

- Minimally invasive procedures are becoming more widely used for the management of upper and lower urinary tract uroliths in cats and dogs.
- Prevention strategies based on stone analysis results should be instituted following urolith removal to limit morbidity and mortality associated with stone recurrence.
- Operator training, careful patient evaluation, and case selection are essential to maximize treatment outcome and limit complications.

INTRODUCTION

Urolithiasis is defined as the formation of uroliths in the urinary tract. Extensive research has been directed at better understanding promotors of stone formation to develop targeted treatment and prevention strategies. In the presence of favorable conditions, urine supersaturation with ionic components of a particular stone type leads to crystal formation, aggregation and growth, and stone formation. Supersaturation of urine is primarily influenced by intrinsic patient factors, certain disease states, water balance, diet, urine pH, the presence of inhibitors of crystallization, aggregation and growth, as well as the presence of a scaffolding matrix.[1–4]

In human medicine, urolithiasis constitutes a health care problem in both adults and children, with a prevalence that is growing every year.[5,6] Considerable focus has been directed toward better understanding risk factors and establishing preventive strategies to improve outcome and reduce stone recurrence in these patients. Moreover, the morbidity and mortality associated with treatment of uroliths have decreased significantly with technical advancements that have led to a shift from open surgery to minimally invasive procedures. Minimally invasive techniques, such as shockwave

Disclosure: The author discloses no conflict of interest.
Department of Clinical Studies, School of Veterinary Medicine, University of Pennsylvania, 3900 Spruce Street, PA 19104, USA
E-mail address: clea@upenn.edu

lithotripsy, ureteroscopy, and percutaneous nephrolithotomy, are now standard of care techniques that constitute primary treatment options recommended by the American Urological Association and European Association of Urology for the management of stone disease in adult and pediatric patients.[7,8]

Following a similar trend, stone management has greatly evolved in veterinary medicine over the past decades, in part because of a better understanding of stone disease in cats and dogs, availability of better diagnostic tools, and also because of the adaptation and application of minimally invasive techniques used in human medicine to small animal patients. The American College of Veterinary Internal Medicine (ACVIM) guidelines for the treatment of uroliths in cats and dogs reflect modern techniques that prioritize the use of minimally invasive procedures with an emphasis on prevention strategies to limit stone morbidity and mortality.[9]

This article reviews minimally invasive techniques used in the management of upper urinary tract and lower urinary tract uroliths. The use of ureteral stenting and subcutaneous ureteral bypass devices for the management of benign ureteral obstructions is covered in Matthew W. Beal's article, "Interventional Management of Urethral Obstructions," in this issue.

UPPER URINARY TRACT UROLITHS

Calcium oxalate uroliths constitute approximately 90% of all nephroliths and ureteroliths in cats.[10,11] They also represent the most frequent type of upper urinary tract stones identified in dogs. A much higher incidence of struvite uroliths exists in this species, with a prevalence ranging between 20% and 30% of all nephroliths and ureteroliths.[12] These differences in stone composition are important to consider when making treatment and prevention recommendations. In canine and feline patients, most nephroliths seem to remain clinically silent and do not necessitate interventions.[9,13] Ross and colleagues[13] evaluated their long-term effects in cats with International Renal Interest Society stage II and III chronic kidney disease for a period of up to 2 years and found no significant impact of nephrolithiasis on disease progression and mortality. However, some nephroliths do become problematic and lead to complications such as urine flow obstruction with hydronephrosis or ureteropelvic junction obstruction, renal parenchyma compression caused by urolith growth, and discomfort, or may act as a nidus for infection, and they can be responsible for recurrent urinary tract infections. In such cases, medical dissolution or stone removal via minimally invasive techniques should be considered.[9,14] The ACVIM consensus recommendations on the treatment of uroliths in small animals recommends medical dissolution for the treatment of nonobstructive struvite nephroliths and ureteroliths. When obstructive, upper urinary tract struvite uroliths first need to be bypassed via ureteral stenting to relieve the obstruction and also allow medicated urine to reach and bathe the stone and for debris to be cleared.[9,14–17] The treatment of cystine and purine nephroliths or ureteroliths should be determined on a case-by-case basis and dissolution attempted when deemed appropriate.[9] Surgical interventions for the management of nephroliths, such as nephrotomy and pyelotomy, have largely been replaced by minimally invasive procedures adapted from human to veterinary patients, like endoscopic nephrolithotomy and extracorporeal shockwave lithotripsy (ESWL). Ureteral stent placement and subcutaneous ureteral bypass devices are used for the treatment of obstructive ureteroliths, and are discussed elsewhere in this issue. The reader should refer to the ACVIM small animal consensus recommendations on the treatment and prevention of uroliths in dogs and cats[9] for a comprehensive review of these recommendations.

Extracorporeal Shockwave Lithotripsy

ESWL was introduced in the early 1980s and has become a standard of care treatment modality for management of upper urinary tract urolithiasis in human medicine. It consists of the generation of high-energy shockwaves by a lithotripter that are transmitted to the patient and allow fragmentation of uroliths. First-generation lithotripters relied on water for acoustic wave transmission and required immersion of the patient and the head of the lithotripter in a water bath. Newer-generation lithotripters have a dry shockwave delivery head, which eliminates the need to immerse the patient in water, and use a water-filled cushion with a silicon membrane for shockwave transmission to the patient.[14,18] Air pockets between the cushion and patient significantly reduce acoustic energy transmission. They have been shown to deflect up to 99% of shockwaves and need to be avoided to minimize dissipation of energy.[19] Using fluoroscopic or ultrasonographic guidance, the urolith is located and the lithotripter focusing system used to direct the shockwaves to the desired target zone. In human pediatric patients, a mean of 2000 shockwaves are delivered per treatment.[8,20,21] Stone fragmentation occurs secondary to mechanical and dynamic forces generated by the shockwaves. These forces have been demonstrated to also cause damage to the vascular endothelium and renal parenchyma as well as adjacent tissues[22,23] with no evidence of long-term morbidity or effect on renal function.[8,23–25] Short-term complications are uncommon and often self-limiting and may include cutaneous bruising, renal hematoma, hematuria, cardiac arrhythmias, and pancreatitis. Ureteral obstruction caused by a stone fragment is also a risk of ESWL.[8,23,26–28] Successful fragmentation and clearance of upper urinary tract uroliths is affected by stone size. In pediatric patients, stone-free rate is affected by stone size with a success rate of approximately 90% for stones measuring less than 1 cm, as opposed to only 60% for stones measuring more than 2 cm after 1 treatment.[8,20,21]

In veterinary medicine, ESWL is recommended for the treatment of problematic nephroliths and ureteroliths measuring less than or equal to 1.5 cm in diameter in dogs. In cases of obstructive ureteroliths, the obstruction must be relieved via ureteral stenting before performing ESWL in an effort to minimize loss of renal function. Placement of a double pigtail ureteral stent in patients with stones measuring more than 1 to 1.5 cm in diameter may be considered before ESWL to allow passive ureteral dilation and reduce the risks of ureteral obstruction by larger stone fragments.[8,29,30] The stone-free rate following ESWL in human patients is not improved by stenting and short-term complications such as discomfort, hematuria, and impaired quality of life have been described with the placement of ureteral stents before the procedure.[31] However, they are advantageous in reducing the incidence of Steinstrasse (stone street), which is the accumulation of stone fragments in the ureter following ESWL and can lead to ureteral obstruction. This condition is encountered more commonly following treatment of larger stones.[32,33] Based on human guidelines, antibiotic prophylaxis is not required for ESWL unless the patient is bacteriuric or the stones are infected.[34] Therefore, a urinalysis and urine culture is recommended before treatment. Patients with a positive culture should receive proper antibiotic therapy based on sensitivity results. ESWL requires general anesthesia to ensure proper patient positioning and limit patient movement. Hair is clipped to limit air bubble entrapment in the fur and allow proper coupling between the patient and the head of the lithotripter. Fluoroscopic and/or ultrasonographic guidance is used for stone localization to position the patient so that the urolith is located within the focal spot of the targeting system (**Fig. 1**). Shockwaves are delivered to induce gradual stone fragmentation. Regular fluoroscopic/ultrasonographic evaluations of the position of the urolith and

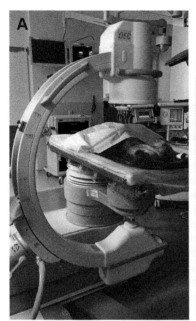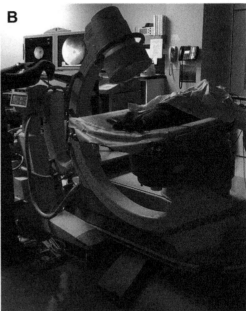

Fig. 1. ESWL in a dog. (*A*) The hair is clipped and the patient placed on the water cushion to ensure proper coupling. (*B*) The nephrolith is positioned in the center of the target zone using fluoroscopy.

adjustments of the focal spot contribute to treatment outcome.[34] Success also depends on the type of lithotripter, stone size, location, composition, and treatment delivered.[14,34] The treatment delivered is influenced by several factors, including pulse energy, shock number, and shock frequency.[35] The shockwave energy is initially set at a low voltage and is progressively increased during treatment (stepwise power ramping). This practice has been demonstrated to lead to greater stone fragmentation compared with protocols using constant output voltage and to better outcomes in some studies.[34–36] During treatment, lower shockwave frequency (60 shockwaves/min) is preferred because of its association with improved outcome and reduced tissue damage compared with a high shock frequency (120 shockwaves/min).[37,38] No consensus for the number of shockwaves delivered has been established in veterinary medicine, but between 1000 and 3500 shocks are commonly used for urolith fragmentation.[39] Fragments around 1 mm are usually generated and move down the ureter and into the bladder over the course of a few weeks. Following the procedure, patients are often hospitalized on intravenous fluids for 24 to 48 hours to promote fluid diuresis and fragment passage to the urinary bladder. Patients with ureteral stents are often discharged sooner because of the decreased risk of a ureteral obstruction post-ESWL, suspected to be caused by passive ureteral dilation following ureteral stent placement. Abdominal radiographs are obtained 24 hours and 1 month after the procedure to look for evidence of residual fragments (**Fig. 2**). Ultrasonography can also be used to evaluate the kidneys for pyelectasia and the presence of fragments that may be too small to be visible on radiographs or that are radiolucent. Similar to the complications reported in human medicine, cutaneous bruising, renal hematoma, hematuria, arrhythmias, pancreatitis, and development of a ureteral obstruction are possible complications in dogs.[14] ESWL is contraindicated in patients with uncontrolled urinary tract

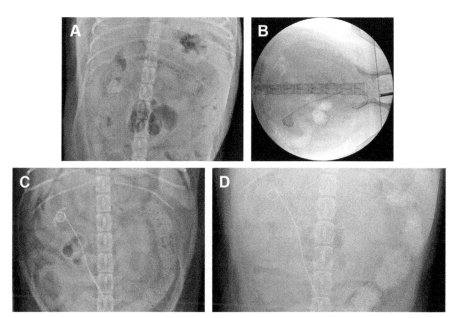

Fig. 2. Imaging performed before and after ESWL in a dog with recurrent urinary tract infections caused by an infected right-sided nephrolith. (*A*) Large right-sided nephrolith. (*B*) Double pigtail right ureteral stent placed before ESWL to prevent development of a ureteral obstruction following stone fragmentation. (*C*) At 24 hours post-ESWL, persistent but improved right nephrolith. (*D*) At 3 weeks post-ESWL, no radiographic evidence of right-sided nephrolith.

infections, coagulation disorders, anatomic obstruction distal to the stone, and in pregnant individuals.[34] ESWL has been used to treat a few cases of nephroliths and/or ureteroliths in cats. However, it is not considered a treatment of choice in this species because of the high risk of ureteral obstruction post-ESWL caused by the small size of their ureters and the size of the stone fragments produced.[14] ESWL is very successful for the treatment of nephroliths and ureteroliths in dogs, with a success rate of approximately 85% and 80%, respectively. Approximately 15% to 30% of patients require additional ESWL treatments to achieve a stone-free state.[14] However, studies evaluating ESWL for the treatment of nephroliths and ureteroliths in dogs are very sparse and data representing stone-free rates, complications, and overall outcome following this procedure remain limited. Stone recurrence is an important factor to consider when managing patients with uroliths, and prevention strategies should be instituted based on the guidelines published by the ACVIM.[9]

Endoscopic Nephrolithotomy

In human patients, endoscopic nephrolithotomy (ENL) is the treatment of choice for nephroliths measuring greater than or equal to 2 cm and for complex nephroliths (staghorn calculi).[34] It has greatly evolved since its introduction, with refinement of the technique and the development of smaller and high-performance instruments. During this procedure, intracorporeal lithotripsy of the nephrolith is performed under fluoroscopic guidance. Compared with ESWL, ENL offers a higher stone-free rate, reduced retreatment rate, and its success is less affected by stone composition and density.[40–42] Cystine stones break into larger fragments and require an increased number of shocks to achieve adequate fragmentation during ESWL, and are considered ESWL resistant.[43] This intervention is more invasive than ESWL, has a higher morbidity rate, and requires longer postoperative hospitalization.[41] Complication rates of 21.3% and 20.5% over a 1-year period were reported in more than 1000 percutaneous ENLs performed in UK centers and in 5724 patients undergoing percutaneous ENL in 96 centers worldwide, respectively.[44] Complications reported for this procedure include fever, bleeding, the need for blood transfusions, sepsis, urinary leakage, and problems associated with residual stones.[40,44] Endoscopic nephrolithotomy has been proved to preserve renal function.[45,46] It also seems to be safe in patients with chronic kidney disease, with a reported improvement of renal function by 10% post-ENL.[47]

In veterinary medicine ENL is practiced by a limited number of highly trained specialists. This procedure is reserved for the treatment of nephroliths in cats and for the treatment of nephroliths that are too large for ESWL in dogs.[9] It is performed percutaneously or surgically assisted, the latter allowing closure of the renal access point. When performed percutaneously, a nephrostomy tube is needed during the time required for healing of the renal access point.

The initial step involves placement of a renal access needle using fluoroscopic and/or ultrasonographic guidance, following a tract through the kidney that allows shortest and most direct access to the nephrolith.[48] A pyeloureterogram is performed under fluoroscopy to confirm positioning of the renal access needle. An angled-tip hydrophilic guidewire is then advanced into the collecting system, down the ureter, into the bladder, and out the urethra, resulting in through-and-through access. Renal tract dilation is then performed to open the renal parenchyma and allow subsequent passage of the access sheath through which the nephroscope is advanced. Various methods of renal tract dilation have been described.[34] With the renal access sheath in place, nephroscopy and nephrolithotomy are performed. Lithotripsy, using an ultrasonic lithotrite or the holmium:yttrium-aluminum-garnet (Hol:YAG) laser, is used to fragment the stone.[14,48] When all stone fragments are removed from the collecting system, a retrograde pyeloureterogram is performed to ensure no stones have traveled down the ureter, and a double pigtail ureteral stent is placed to span the renal pelvis, ureter, and bladder. Because of the small ureteral diameter and the complications associated with prophylactic ureteral stenting in cats, ureteral stenting following ENL in this species is not performed. Following ENL, a nephrostomy tube is placed if performed percutaneously or the renal tract is sutured closed if performed surgically assisted.[14] One of the most common problems encountered perioperatively in humans following ENL are infectious complications, such as urinary tract infection and urosepsis. Despite negative voided urine cultures obtained preoperatively, studies have reported positive cultures of urine collected from the pelvis or from stones removed intraoperatively in 25% or more of human patients.[49] In the absence of guidelines in veterinary medicine, human guidelines should be followed and include performing a urinalysis and urine culture before treatment. Patients with a positive culture should receive proper antibiotic therapy based on urine sensitivity results. The administration of perioperative prophylactic antibiotics is also recommended, because it has been shown to reduce the rate of infectious complications in humans.[34,40,49] Following the procedure, patients are hospitalized and monitored for evidence of uroabdomen and sepsis concerns. Ultrasonography is performed to evaluate the urinary tract following the procedure and look for evidence of urine leakage. Radiographs can also be performed to look for the presence of stone fragments in the urinary tract. Similar to the complications reported in human medicine, urine leakage and blood loss are among the most common complications reported in veterinary patients.[14] Berent and colleagues[14] described the use of ENL for the treatment of complicated nephroliths in 9 dogs and 1 cat. Their data showed a preoperative median creatinine level of 1.3 mg/dL (range 0.8–9.1 mg/dL) and of 1.1 mg/dL (range 0.6–6.1 mg/dL) 3 months postoperatively. A stone-free state was achieved in 92% of renal units. Rate of complication (3 out of 9) was similar to what is reported in the human literature, and all were easily managed. Based on these results, endoscopic nephrolithotomy was reported to be safe in dogs and cats for the treatment of complicated nephroliths. The stone-free rate achieved in this study was also similar to the success rate reported in the human literature, in which stone-free rates around 90% have been reported. It is important to note that various definitions have been used to describe stone-free rates following ENL in humans. Many exclude clinically insignificant fragments, which are residual fragments less than or equal to 4 mm in diameter, when reporting stone-free rates. Therefore, the stone-free rates reported depend on the imaging modality used, when imaging is performed post-ENL, and the definition of stone-free used. A study evaluating the stone-free rate after percutaneous ENL in human patients reported a true stone-free rate of 55%. However, nearly 85% of patients had a stone-free rate when clinically insignificant fragments were not included in calculation, which correlates with previous studies.[50] Studies evaluating ENL for the treatment of nephroliths are sparse and data representing stone-free rates, complications, and overall outcome following this procedure remain limited. Stone recurrence is an important factor to consider when managing patients with uroliths and prevention strategies should be instituted based on the guidelines published by the ACVIM.[9]

LOWER URINARY TRACT UROLITHS

Calcium oxalate and struvite uroliths are the most commonly identified types of lower urinary tract stones in dogs and cats.[10,12] Patients may be asymptomatic or exhibit clinical signs, such as hematuria, pollakiuria, and stranguria. In some cases, they present with a urethral obstruction and require emergency intervention. Medical dissolution should be considered in cases of nonobstructive bladder stones when radiographic findings, urinalysis, and urine culture results are suggestive of a composition of struvite.[9] Several studies have demonstrated the effectiveness and safety of dissolution diets as part of the management strategies for the treatment of struvite stones in cats and dogs.[1,51] Medical dissolution should also be considered for the management of urate and cystine cystoliths.

In the past, cystotomy has been the treatment of choice for lower urinary tract stone removal. However, with incomplete urolith removal[52] in some cases following cystotomy, a reported risk of suture-induced stone formation of up to 9%,[53] and the high recurrence rate of certain types of stones, removal is only indicated for cases of cystoliths associated with clinical signs or with the potential to cause a urinary obstruction or cases of urethral stones.[9] Removal of these stones with minimally invasive techniques is recommended by the ACVIM consensus recommendations on the treatment of uroliths in dogs and cats.[9] Techniques described include voiding urohydropropulsion, cystoscopic-guided basket retrieval, cystoscopic-guided laser lithotripsy, and percutaneous cystolithotomy (PCCL). These techniques have the potential complication of bladder rupture and therefore all patients undergoing one of these procedures should have a negative urine culture before the procedure. Voiding urohydropropulsion has been described as a simple and effective method for removal of small cystoliths in dogs and female cats. Using this technique, cystoliths less than or equal to

3 mm can generally be removed in female cats and in male dogs, and those that are less than or equal to 4 to 5 mm can be voided from female dogs.[9] However, the largest stone size removed has rarely been reported and these guidelines may vary based on the size of the patient and the stone shape. This technique is not indicated in male cats. Hematuria is common following the procedure and typically self-resolves within a few hours to days.[54] Other possible complications include urethral obstruction, and incomplete stone removal. If voiding urohydropropulsion is not indicated for a given patient, other minimally invasive options, including cystoscopic-guided basket retrieval and laser lithotripsy, and PCCL should be considered.

Regardless of the technique used, all stones removed should be submitted for analysis to allow optimal prevention strategies to be implemented based on stone composition. The reader should refer to the ACVIM small animal consensus recommendations on the treatment and prevention of uroliths in dogs and cats[9] for a comprehensive review of these recommendations.

Cystoscopic-Guided Basket Retrieval

Cystoscopic-guided basket retrieval (**Fig. 3**) involves transurethral cystoscopic evaluation of the lower urinary tract followed by urolith basket retrieval. This technique can be used in dogs and female cats. In this technique, basket retrieval devices are used to grasp stones that are too big to be expelled via voiding urohydropropulsion but that are smaller than the urethral diameter. This technique is also commonly used following laser lithotripsy (described later). Various sizes and shapes of basket retrieval devices

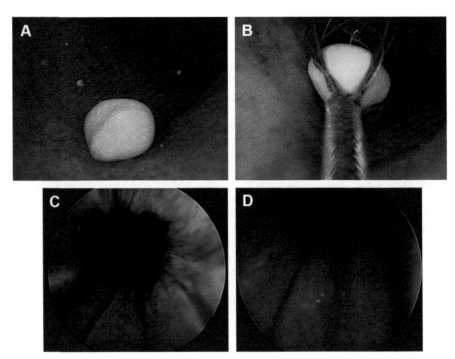

Fig. 3. Transurethral cystoscopic-guided urolith basket retrieval. (*A*) The urolith is localized cystoscopically. (*B*) The basket is passed via the working channel of the cystoscope and used to grasp the stone. (*C*) Appearance of the urethra before stone removal. (*D*) Appearance of the urethra following stone removal with some inflammation noted.

are available. When the stones to be removed via basket retrieval are localized, a basket is introduced within the working channel of the rigid or flexible cystoscope and advanced until it is exteriorized at the tip of the cystoscope. When in the closed position, the basket is compressed under a protective sheath and can be passed via the working channel. When in the opened position, the basket is fully deployed and can be used to encircle stones. Once a urolith is grasped, the basket is closed and gently pulled back to the tip of the cystoscope, and the cystoscope and basket retrieval device are simultaneously removed from the lower urinary tract. It is important not to force the removal of stones that are too big to pass through the urethra, which could lead to urethral tears. Each stone removed via basket retrieval involves the introduction and removal of the cystoscope into the lower urinary tract, with each stone contacting and potentially traumatizing the urethral mucosa on removal. Therefore, urolith basket removal is not recommended in cases in which there is a large number of stones present because of the repeated trauma to the urethral mucosa as stones are being removed. Percutaneous cystolithotomy should be considered in these cases to avoid urethral trauma. Cystoscopic-guided stone basket retrieval is highly successful for the removal of uroliths with proper case selection.

Cystoscopic-Guided Laser Lithotripsy

The word laser is an acronym for light amplification by stimulated emission of radiation. Laser lithotripsy is widely used for intracorporeal lithotripsy in human medicine. In laser lithotripsy, light is emitted and causes stone fragmentation via generation of photothermal energy.[55,56] Various laser types have been developed, but the Hol:YAG is more commonly used. The Hol:YAG laser has a wavelength of 2.1 μm with a pulsed activity.[56] Its energy is absorbed by fluid and can therefore be used in close proximity to the mucosal wall without causing significant damage, including tight locations within the urethra.[39,55]

Laser lithotripsy (**Fig. 4**) is a minimally invasive technique used in veterinary medicine for the fragmentation of stones that are larger than the urethral diameter. It involves transurethral cystoscopic evaluation of the lower urinary tract followed by intracorporeal laser lithotripsy in which uroliths are fragmented into smaller pieces and removed via voiding urohydropropulsion and/or basket retrieval. This treatment modality is indicated in dogs and female cats. It can be used to fragment uroliths of any type located in the urinary bladder or urethra.[57] Studies have reported complete removal of uroliths in 83% to 100% of female and 81% to 87% of male dogs following laser lithotripsy with proper case selection.[58,59] When laser time was evaluated, laser time was shorter in dogs with urethroliths than in dogs with cystoliths.[58] Moreover, when the rate of complete urolith removal was evaluated based on stone location, complete removal was documented in all dogs with urethroliths as opposed to 79% of dogs with cystoliths, and 76% of dogs with a combination of cystoliths and urethroliths.[59]

Female cats and dogs are generally positioned in dorsal recumbency and male dogs in dorsal or lateral recumbency for cystoscopy and laser lithotripsy. Following standard aseptic preparation, transurethral cystoscopic evaluation of the lower urinary tract is performed. When the stone to be fragmented is localized, the laser fiber is introduced within the working channel of the rigid or flexible cystoscope and advanced until it is exteriorized at the tip of the cystoscope. It can be used in both rigid and flexible cystoscopes. During lithotripsy, the laser fiber is advanced until it touches the stone, avoiding contact with the urinary bladder or urethral mucosa. Fluid irrigation with sterile saline is used to maintain visualization of the urolith and to dissipate heat near the tip of the laser fiber. Following stone fragmentation, voiding urohydropropulsion and/or basket retrieval are used to remove the smaller fragments.

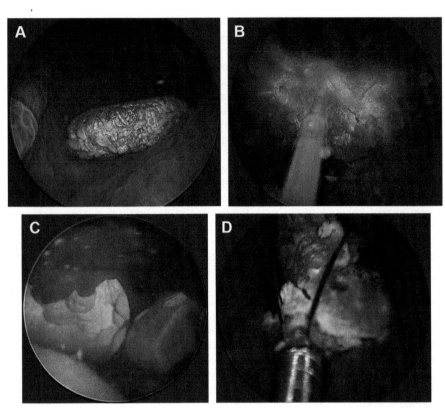

Fig. 4. Transurethral cystoscopic-guided laser lithotripsy. (*A*) The urolith is localized. (*B*) The Hol:YAG fiber is passed via the working channel of the cystoscope and advanced until it is in contact with the stone for laser lithotripsy. (*C*) Stone fragments following laser lithotripsy. (*D*) The fragments are removed via voiding urohydropropulsion or basket retrieval.

This technique is safe and effective for minimally invasive removal of cystoliths and urethroliths in dogs and female cats. Complications associated with this procedure typically occur during or within 24 hours of the procedure. Most commonly, hematuria and the need for an indwelling urinary catheter caused by urethral swelling causing a partial or complete urinary tract obstruction have been reported.[58,59] Others include perforation of the bladder wall during voiding urohydropropulsion, urethral tear, and urethral stricture.[58,60] Proper case selection is important when considering intracorporeal laser lithotripsy and the patient should be big enough to allow easy passage into the urinary bladder and maneuvering of the cystoscope. Moreover, this technique should not be recommended in animals with a large stone burden or large stones because of concerns for urethral trauma and excessive anesthesia time relative to other treatment strategies.

Percutaneous Cystolithotomy

PCCL is a minimally invasive procedure that has been used for the management of bladder stones in human pediatric patients as an alternative to open surgery. Their small urethral diameter precludes the use of transurethral treatment modalities in this subset of patients.[61] Similarly, many small animal patients have a small urethral diameter, preventing the use of voiding urohydropropulsion, transurethral laser lithotripsy, and/or urolith basket retrieval. This technique (**Fig. 5**) was adapted to veterinary patients and can be performed in both cats and dogs, of any sex or size. PCCL allows the removal of stones located both in the bladder and the urethra.

PCCL was described in 23 dogs and 4 cats (2 males, 2 females) with bladder and urethral stones. It was performed in patients weighing between 1.8 to 42.6 kg in whom 1 to more than 35 uroliths had been identified. All patients were discharged within 24 hours following the procedure and no postoperative complications were reported.[62] Some of the advantages of this procedure include the ability to fully distend the bladder to inspect the bladder and urethra for the presence of residual uroliths while causing minimal hemorrhage, inflammation, trauma, and limiting bladder manipulation.[60,62] In this study, there was a 3.7% (1 out of 27 patients) incidence of incomplete stone removal, as shown on recheck radiographs following PCCL.[62]

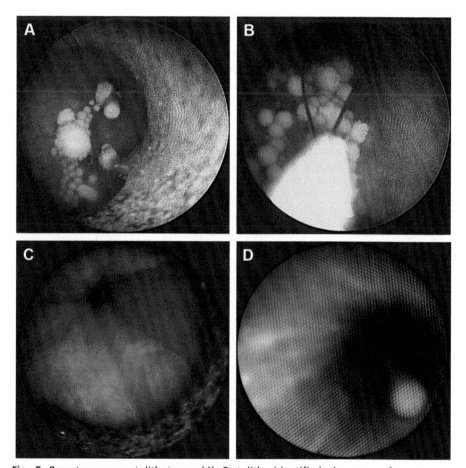

Fig. 5. Percutaneous cystolithotomy. (*A*) Cystoliths identified via antegrade cystoscopy through the cannula. (*B*) The basket retrieval device is passed via the working channel of the cystoscope and used to grasp the stones. (*C*) Following stone removal, the urinary bladder is inspected to ensure all cystoliths have been removed. (*D*) Antegrade urethroscopy to ensure all urethroliths have been removed. (*Courtesy of* Jeffrey J. Runge, DVM, Philadelphia, PA.)

For PCCL, patients are positioned in dorsal recumbency and are aseptically prepared. A red rubber urinary catheter is passed into the urethra and bladder. A small midline skin incision (1.5–2 cm) and abdominal incision (1–1.5 cm) are made over the apex of the bladder. The bladder is grabbed and held at the level of the incision with the aid of stay sutures. A small stab incision is made into the bladder and a threaded cannula is advanced into the incision. A rigid cystoscope is then passed through the cannula to allow identification of the uroliths and evaluation of the bladder mucosa. The cystoscope is removed and the uroliths are suctioned while saline is simultaneously being infused through the red rubber catheter. For larger uroliths, retrieval of the stones via the cannula using a basket retrieval device can be used.

When all uroliths have been removed, a cystoscope is used to perform a final inspection of the bladder. A flexible cystoscope is then advanced into the urethra as the red rubbed is removed while infusing saline to ensure retrograde flushing of any residual urethroliths. The bladder, abdominal, and skin incisions are closed using standard technique.[60,62]

This technique is commonly used for the minimally invasive removal of cystoliths and urethroliths in cats and dogs. Possible complications associated with this procedure include urine leakage, incomplete stone removal, and other complications reported with cystotomies.[60]

SUMMARY

Minimally invasive procedures are becoming more commonly used for the management of uroliths in cats and dogs. These procedures should be performed by trained operators. Careful patient evaluation and case selection is essential to maximize treatment outcome and limit complications.

REFERENCES

1. Bartges JW, Callens AJ. Urolithiasis. Vet Clin North Am Small Anim Pract 2015;45: 747–68.
2. Bushinsky DA, Monk RD. Nephrolithiasis and nephrocalcinosis. In: Johnson RJ, Feehally J, Floege J, editors. Comprehensive clinical nephrology. 5th edition. Philadelphia: Elsevier Saunders; 2015. p. 688–702.
3. Chew DJ, DiBartola SP, Schenck PA. Urolithasis. In: Chew DJ, DiBartola SP, Schenck PA, editors. Canine and Feline nephrology and urology. 2nd edition. St Louis (MO): Elsevier Saunders; 2011. p. 272–305.
4. Kaiser J, Stěpánková K, Kořistková T, et al. Determination of the cause of selected canine urolith formation by advanced analytical methods. J Small Anim Pract 2012;53:646–51.
5. Kirkali Z, Rasooly R, Star RA, et al. Urinary stone disease: progress, status, and needs. Urology 2012;86:651–3.
6. Tasian GE, Copelovitch L. Evaluation and medical management of kidney stones in children. J Urol 2014;192:1329–36.
7. Assimos D, Krambeck A, Miller NL, et al. Surgical management of stones: American Urological Association/Endourological Society Guideline. 2016. Available at: http://www.auanet.org/guidelines/surgical-management-of-stones-(aua/endourological-society-guideline-2016. Accessed January 29, 2018.
8. Tekgül S, Dogan HS, Kocvara R, et al. Pediatric urology. 2017. Available at: http://uroweb.org/guideline/paediatric-urology/. Accessed January 29, 2018.

9. Lulich JP, Berent AC, Adams LG, et al. ACVIM small animal consensus recommendations on the treatment and prevention of uroliths in dogs and cats. J Vet Intern Med 2016;30:1564–74.

10. Cannon AB, Westropp JL, Ruby AL, et al. Evaluation of trends in urolith composition in cats: 5,230 cases (1985-2004). J Am Vet Med Assoc 2007;231:570–6.

11. Kyles AE, Hardie EM, Wooden BG, et al. Management and outcome of cats with ureteral calculi: 153 cases (1984-2002). J Am Vet Med Assoc 2005;226:937–44.

12. Low WW, Uhl JM, Kass PH, et al. Evaluation of trends in urolith composition and characteristics of dogs with urolithiasis: 25,499 cases (1985-2006). J Am Vet Med Assoc 2010;236:193–200.

13. Ross SJ, Osborne CA, Lekcharoensuk C, et al. A case-control study of the effects of nephrolithiasis in cats with chronic kidney disease. J Am Vet Med Assoc 2007; 230:1854–9.

14. Berent AC, Adams LG. Interventional management of complicated nephrolithiasis. In: Weisse C, Berent A, editors. Veterinary image-guided interventions. Ames (IA): Wiley-Blackwell; 2015. p. 289–300.

15. Berent AC, Weisse CW, Todd K, et al. Technical and clinical outcomes of ureteral stenting in cats with benign ureteral obstruction: 69 cases (2006-2010). J Am Vet Med Assoc 2014;244:559–76.

16. Kuntz JA, Berent AC, Weisse CW, et al. Double pigtail ureteral stenting and renal pelvic lavage for renal-sparing treatment of obstructive pyonephrosis in dogs: 13 cases (2008-2012). J Am Vet Med Assoc 2015;246:216–25.

17. Palm CA, Culp WTN. Nephroureteral obstructions – the use of stents and ureteral bypass systems for renal decompression. Vet Clin North Am Small Anim Pract 2016;46:1183–92.

18. McClain PD, Lange JN, Assimos DG. Optimizing shock wave lithotripsy: a comprehensive review. Rev Urol 2013;15:49–60.

19. Pishchalnikov YA, Neucks JS, VonDerHaar RJ, et al. Air pockets trapped during routine coupling in dry head lithotripsy can significantly decrease the delivery of shockwave energy. J Urol 2006;176:2706–10.

20. Raza A, Turna B, Smith G, et al. Pediatric urolithiasis: 15 years of local experience with minimally invasive endourological management of pediatric calculi. J Urol 2005;174(2):682–5.

21. Muslumanoglu AY, Tefekli A, Sarilar O, et al. Extracorporeal shock wave lithotripsy as first line treatment alternative for urinary tract stones in children: a large scale retrospective analysis. J Urol 2003;170:2405–8.

22. Wood K, Keys T, Mufarrij P, et al. Impact of stone removal on renal function: a review. Rev Urol 2011;13:73–89.

23. Skolarikos A, Alivizatos G, de la Rosette J. Extracorporeal shock wave lithotripsy 25 years later: complications and their prevention. Eur Urol 2006;50:981–90.

24. McLorie GA, Pugach J, Pode D, et al. Safety and efficacy of extracorporeal shock wave lithotripsy in infants. Can J Urol 2003;10:2051–5.

25. Vlajković M, Slavković A, Radovanović M, et al. Long-term functional outcome of kidneys in children with urolithiasis after ESWL treatment. Eur J Pediatr Surg 2002;12:118–23.

26. Drake T, Grivas N, Dabestani S, et al. What are the benefits and harms of ureteroscopy compared with shock-wave lithotripsy in the treatment of upper ureteral stones? A systematic review. Eur Urol 2017;72:772–86.

27. Alzahrani T, Ghiculete D, Pace TK, et al. Changing patient position can eliminate arrhythmias developing during extracorporeal shockwave lithotripsy. J Endourol 2016;30:550–4.

28. McAteer JA, Evan AP. The acute and long-term adverse effects of shockwave lithotripsy. Semin Nephrol 2008;28:200–13.

29. Adams LG, Goldman CK. Extracorporeal shockwave lithotripsy. In: Bartges DJ, Polzin D, editors. Nephrology and urology of small animals. Ames (IA): Blackwell; 2011. p. 340–8.

30. Vachon C, Brisson B, Nykamp S, et al. Passive ureteral dilation and ureteroscopy after ureteral stent placement in five healthy Beagles. Am J Vet Res 2017;78: 381–92.

31. Musa AA. Use of double-J stents prior to extracorporeal shock wave lithotripsy is not beneficial: results of a prospective randomized study. Int Urol Nephrol 2008; 40:19–22.

32. Shen P, Jiang M, Yang J, et al. Use of ureteral stent in extracorporeal shock wave lithotripsy for upper urinary calculi: a systematic review and meta-analysis. J Urol 2011;186:1328–35.

33. Sayed MA, el-Taher AM, Aboul-Ella HA, et al. Steinstrasse after extracorporeal shockwave lithotripsy: aetiology, prevention and management. BJU Int 2001;88: 675–8.

34. Türk C, Neisius A, Petrik A, et al. Urolithiasis. 2017. Available at: http://uroweb. org/guideline/urolithiasis/. Accessed February 1, 2018.

35. Demirci D, Sofikerim M, Yalçin E, et al. Comparison of conventional and step-wise shockwave lithotripsy in management of urinary calculi. J Endourol 2007;21: 1407–10.

36. Maloney ME, Marguet CG, Zhou Y, et al. Progressive increase of lithotripter output produces better in-vivo stone comminution. J Endourol 2006;20:603–6.

37. Kang DH, Cho KS, Ham WS, et al. Comparison of high, intermediate, and low frequency shock wave lithotripsy for urinary tract stone disease: systematic review and network meta-analysis. PLoS One 2016;11:e0158661.

38. Connors BA, Evan AP, Blomgren EP, et al. Extracorporeal shock wave lithotripsy at 60 shock waves/min reduces renal injury in a porcine model. BJU Int 2009;104: 1004–8.

39. Berent AC. Interventional Urology: endourology in small animal veterinary medicine. Vet Clin North Am Small Anim Pract 2015;45:825–55.

40. Assimos D, Krambeck A, Miller NL, et al. Surgical management of stones: AUA/ Endourology society guideline. 2016. Available at: http://www.auanet.org/ guidelines/surgical-management-of-stones-(aua/endourological-society-guideline-2016. Accessed February 2, 2018.

41. Srisubat A, Potisat S, Lojanapiwat B, et al. Extracorporeal shock wave lithotripsy (ESWL) versus percutaneous nephrolithotomy (PCNL) or retrograde intrarenal surgery (RIRS) for kidney stones. Cochrane Database Syst Rev 2014;11:4–43.

42. Donaldson JF, Lardas M, Scrimgeour D, et al. Systematic review and meta-analysis of the clinical effectiveness of shock wave lithotripsy, retrograde intrarenal surgery, and percutaneous nephrolithotomy for lower-pole renal stones. Eur Urol 2015;67:612–6.

43. Katz G, Shapiro A, Lencovsky Z, et al. Place of extracorporeal shock-wave lithotripsy (ESWL) in management of cystine calculi. Urology 1990;36:124–8.

44. Ghani KR, Andonian S, Bultitude M, et al. Percutaneous nephrolithotomy: update, trends, and future directions. Eur Urol 2016;70:382–96.

45. Pérez-Fentes D, Cortés J, Gude F, et al. Does percutaneous nephrolithotomy and its outcomes can have an impact on renal function? Quantitative analysis using SPECT-CT DMSA. Urolithiasis 2014;42:461–7.

46. Ünsal A, Koca G, Resorlu B, et al. Effect of percutaneous nephrolithotomy and tract dilatation methods on renal function: assessment by quantitative single-photon emission computer tomography of technectium-99m-dimercaptosuccinic acid update by the kidneys. J Endourol 2010;24:1497–502.

47. Jones P, Aboumarzouk OM, Zelhof B, et al. Percutaneous nephrolithotomy in patients with chronic kidney disease: efficacy and safety. Urology 2017;108:1–6.

48. Smaldone MC, Docimo SG, Ost M. Contemporary surgical management of pediatric urolithiasis. Urol Clin North Am 2010;37:253–67.

49. Wollin DA, Preminger GM. Percutaneous nephrolithotomy: complications and how to deal with them. Urolithiasis 2018;46:87–97.

50. Emmott AS, Brotherhood HL, Paterson RF, et al. Complications, re-intervention rates, and natural history of residual stone fragments after percutaneous nephrolithotomy. J Endourol 2018;32:28–32.

51. Lulich JP, Kruger JM, MacLeay JM, et al. Efficacy of two commercially available, low-magnesium, urine-acidifying dry foods for the dissolution of struvite uroliths in cats. J Am Vet Med Assoc 2016;243:1147–53.

52. Grant DC, Harper TAM, Werre SR. Frequency of incomplete urolith removal, complications, and diagnostic imaging following cystotomy for removal or uroliths from the lower urinary tract in dogs: 128 cases (1994-2006). J Am Vet Med Assoc 2010;236:736–66.

53. Appel SL, Lefebvre SL, Houston DM, et al. Evaluation of risk factors associated with suture-nidus cystoliths in dogs and cats: 176 cases (1999-2006). J Am Vet Med Assoc 2008;233:1889–95.

54. Lulich JP, Osborne CA, Carlson M, et al. Nonsurgical removal of urocystoliths in dogs and cats by voiding urohydropropulsion. J Am Vet Med Assoc 1993;203:660–3.

55. Scotland KB, Krozack T, Pace KT, et al. Stone technology: intracorporeal lithotripters. World J Urol 2017;35:1347–51.

56. Dolowy L, Krajewski W, Dembowski J, et al. The role of lasers in modern urology. Cent European J Urol 2015;68:175–82.

57. Ywnn VM, Davidson EB, Higbee RG, et al. In vitro effects of pulsed holmium laser energy on canine uroliths and porcine cadaveric urethra. Lasers Surg Med 2003;33:243–6.

58. Adams LG, Berent AC, Moore GE, et al. Use of laser lithotripsy for fragmentation of uroliths in dogs: 73 cases (2005-2006). J Am Vet Med Assoc 2008;232:1680–7.

59. Lulich JP, Osborne CA, Albasan H, et al. Efficacy and safety of laser lithotripsy in fragmentation of urocystoliths and urethroliths for removal in dogs. J Am Vet Med Assoc 2009;234:1279–85.

60. Berent AC, Adams LG. Minimally invasive treatment of bladder and urethral stones in dogs and cats. In: Weisse C, Berent A, editors. Veterinary image-guided interventions. Ames (IA): Wiley-Blackwell; 2015. p. 360–72.

61. Agrawal MS, Aron M, Goyal J, et al. Percutaneous suprapubic cystolithotripsy for vesical calculi in children. J Endourol 1999;13:173–5.

62. Runge JJ, Berent AC, Meyhew PD, et al. Transvesicular percutaneous cystolithotomy for the retrieval of cystic and urethral calculi in dogs and cats: 27 cases (2006-2008). J Am Vet Med Assoc 2011;239:344–9.

Interventional Radiology Management of Nonresectable Neoplasia

William T.N. Culp, VMD

KEYWORDS

- Locoregional therapy • Intra-arterial chemotherapy • Embolization
- Chemoembolization • Stent

KEY POINTS

- Image-guidance allows for the performance of alternative techniques in the treatment of nonresectable neoplasia.
- Locoregional therapies can be considered for the treatment of a myriad of tumors; however, extensive understanding of anatomy and available techniques is required.
- Early outcomes associated with the interventional radiology management of nonresectable neoplasia are promising, although further evaluation of long-term outcomes is necessary.

INTRODUCTION

As medical and technological advances occur, it is inevitable that options for the treatment of neoplastic disease will increase. With the availability of evolving, innovative options, it is essential for treating clinicians and owners to work closely together to determine the best diagnostic and therapeutic course of action for a particular patient. It is always important to consider that while "something" can be done, it may not always be in that patient's best interest. With that fact in mind, advances in instrumentation and other technologies using interventional radiology (IR) or more specifically interventional oncology (IO), techniques provide owners with treatment options, especially for the many cases that had no options only a short time ago. Most of these options are considered palliative in nature but have the potential to provide an improved quality of life.

TREATMENT OPTIONS

The major treatment option categories for oncologic disease have not changed much in the last several decades. In general, surgery should be considered whenever

Veterinary Medical Teaching Hospital, University of California-Davis, School of Veterinary Medicine, One Garrod Drive, Davis, CA 95616, USA
E-mail address: wculp@ucdavis.edu

Vet Clin Small Anim 48 (2018) 891–898
https://doi.org/10.1016/j.cvsm.2018.05.007
0195-5616/18/© 2018 Elsevier Inc. All rights reserved.

possible. Depending on tumor type, location, and biological behavior, chemotherapy and radiation therapy may be used in a neoadjuvant or adjuvant setting or as primary treatment modalities. The concept of "nonresectability" is a controversial topic because it is often clinician-dependent. As an example, some surgeons may feel that certain prostatic tumors can be removed with an aggressive prostatectomy approach, whereas others would be reluctant to consider this procedure due to the potential complications or the chance of recurrence. When surgery may be considered a poor option due to tumor location or severity of organ involvement, IO treatment options such as locoregional therapies or stenting can be considered.

ASSESSMENT OF TUMOR RESECTABILITY AND GOALS OF THERAPY

Although patient history, physical examination, and blood work are extremely important in the global assessment of a patient, these do not likely provide significant information about a particular tumor's resectability. Advanced imaging (often beyond ultrasonography) is often needed, and in the author's clinic, this is generally performed with computed tomography (CT) and magnetic resonance imaging (MRI). Although these modalities may not provide a total understanding of a tumor's resectability, and surgery may be required to manipulate the tumor, CT and MRI have several properties that make them useful for preprocedural tumor assessment. First, a general sense of a tumor's location and what adjacent structures/organs are involved can be obtained due to the cross-sectional imaging capacity of these modalities. Second, the vascular supply to tumors can be assessed and mapped, which can be useful for resection or for locoregional vascular therapies. Lastly, CT and MRI are commonly used to determine response to treatment through assessment of tumor size and characteristics before and after treatment.

Luminal patency, or lack thereof, is often best depicted using a real-time imaging modality such as fluoroscopy. Injection of contrast medium while recording fluoroscopic images allows a clinician to determine the location of an obstruction, severity of obstruction (ie, alteration of luminal diameter), and normal luminal size. In addition, it is possible to assess the efficacy of the opening of a malignant luminal obstruction after placement of a stent. In companion animals, malignant luminal obstructions in the urethra, ureter, esophagus, colon, and nasopharynx are often assessed using fluoroscopic imaging combined with the injection of contrast medium.

Although a tumor may be able to be resected in some patients from a surgical prowess standpoint, the removal of a tumor may otherwise compromise an organ and subsequently the patient. An example of this is large liver resections in human patients. In humans, the calculation of functional liver remnant is commonplace and is often performed before a large tumor resection.[1,2] This remnant is measured before a resection to determine whether a patient can tolerate the proposed amount of tissue to be resected in an effort to prevent liver failure secondary to loss of liver tissue. If the remaining liver tissue does not seem to be sufficient for a particular patient, an alternative therapy such as portal vein embolization may be considered before resection in an attempt to generate more functional liver tissue.[1,2] There is a scarcity of clinical data related to this topic in companion animals.

When considering an IO procedure in a case that has a tumor that is considered nonresectable, the goals of treatment should be well defined. Some possible questions to consider are as follows:

Is the IO procedure being used as a primary or adjuvant therapy?
Is the objective to downstage the tumor?
Is the procedure being performed to make the tumor resectable?

Is the procedure designed to act as a "bridge" therapy (ie, control tumor growth while waiting for a more definitive therapy)?

In human patients, these types of questions are crucial because IO techniques have now demonstrated several advances over the last few decades. These treatments include similar local tumor control and survival rates to surgical resection in some settings. These procedures are performed minimally invasively allowing for less postprocedural discomfort and earlier recovery and can be considered neoadjuvantly to make a nonresectable tumor amenable to resection or adjuvantly to reduce the risk of recurrence.[3]

BIOPSY

Image modalities such as ultrasonography, fluoroscopy, and CT can be used to guide biopsy acquisition. In many instances, biopsies are obtained presurgery, but biopsies may also be useful to guide therapy for nonresectable neoplasia. In the author's practice, fluoroscopic-guidance of bone biopsies is pursued regularly to guide placement of the biopsy device (**Fig. 1**). Bone biopsies are often acquired in cases where surgery may not be pursued, such as bony metastatic disease or tumors of bone where resection may not be advisable (eg, plasma cell tumors).

LOCOREGIONAL THERAPIES

When surgical options for tumor removal are either not feasible or not elected, a locoregional therapy can be considered in an attempt to control tumors locally, stimulate tumor necrosis, or palliate clinical signs. Locoregional therapies are broadly categorized into transarterial therapies and ablative therapies. These treatments are generally focused on tumor-specific targeting, either by direct application or by access to the arterial blood supply. Both transarterial and ablative therapies are well established in human medicine, and the use of these treatments in veterinary patients is growing. Ablative therapies are generally used in the treatment of smaller tumors, many of which may also be treated with surgery. However, this treatment modality can also be used to treat metastatic disease or multiple affected areas within an organ.

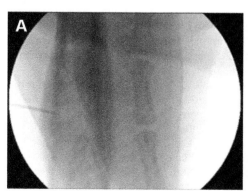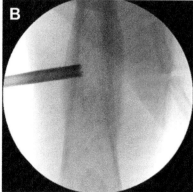

Fig. 1. Fluoroscopic images of a bone biopsy. (*A*) Using fluoroscopic-guidance, a needle is directed at the region of bone that is abnormal. (*B*) After establishing the location and angle needed to obtain the bone from the region of interest using a needle, a bone biopsy device can be used to obtain the sample. Penetration through the cis cortex can be confirmed with fluoroscopy.

Locoregional transarterial therapies use the local delivery of chemotherapy, radiation therapy, or embolic agents to the tumoral blood supply. To perform these procedures, a strong understanding of regional anatomy and imaging interpretation is necessary. It is highly recommended to perform preprocedural imaging assessment of tumors with CT or MRI to identify tumor location and blood supply to allow for a "map" to be created before performing the procedure. Intraprocedure angiography will provide real-time assessment of the direct blood supply to a tumor as well as the velocity of blood flow in that region. In addition, fluoroscopic angiography will help assess a tumor for the presence of vascular shunting, which can occur secondary to the disease process and may complicate or limit the treatment options.

The information regarding fluoroscopic arterial anatomy available to veterinary clinicians interested in performing these procedures is limited. Currently, one report describes the fluoroscopic arterial anatomy of the abdominal organs.[4] This study describes general positioning of the abdominal arterial first order branches and their smaller branches and compares to vertebral positioning to allow for targeting of certain branches with a goal of decreasing contrast medium administration and fluoroscopic time. In addition, understanding the normal abdominal arterial anatomy will improve the chances of being able to identify abnormal anatomy and improve targeting of tumoral blood supply. More work into this area is needed because these procedures are becoming more common for nonresectable tumors.

In general, the transarterial approach is performed through either the carotid or the femoral artery in companion animals. Surgical dissection to the artery is most commonly performed to ensure adequate postoperative hemostasis, although ultrasound-guided percutaneous access is also possible. After arterial access is achieved, a series of wires, sheaths, and catheters are used in coaxial fashion to gain access to the region of interest. The clinicians performing these cases should familiarize themselves with the use of microcatheters and microwires, because these small versions of these instruments have unique properties and challenges but are essential to access most tumor vasculature. In companion animals, the microcatheters generally used are in the range of 1.8 to 2.7 Fr and microwires in the range of 0.010 to 0.014″ in diameter.

Intra-arterial chemotherapy (IAC) has been proposed as an advantageous use of chemotherapy compared with intravenous delivery because of the ability of administering higher doses of chemotherapy directly to a tumor and decreasing potential side effects associated with chemotherapy. The impact of IAC on disease-free interval and survival remains controversial despite much research being focused on the topic in the human medical field.

Althoug a common practice in human patients, IAC administration has been rarely used in veterinary patients but can be considered in cases where surgical resection cannot or will not be pursued. In addition, in humans, IAC is used as a means of tumor margin sterilization or preoperatively with the intent of decreasing the likelihood of postoperative recurrence.[5] These indications have not been pursued in veterinary patients, to the author's knowledge. The administration of IAC was compared with intravenous chemotherapy (IVC) in a recent report of dogs with lower urinary tract carcinoma.[6] In that study, a combination of carboplatin and a nonsteroidal antiinflammatory drug (NSAID) was administered after attempting superselection of the tumoral arterial blood supply in the IAC group. In the IVC group, dogs received carboplatin intravenously and an oral NSAID. The short-term tumor response to IAC was greater than the response to IVC, and dogs receiving IAC were significantly less likely to experience side effects such as anemia, lethargy, and anorexia.[6]

Embolization is the delivery of an embolic agent to a selected blood vessel to cause slowing or cessation of blood flow via vascular occlusion. Embolization is theorized to work by causing necrosis of tumor cells secondary to alteration of blood flow. When embolization is combined with chemotherapy, the procedure is called chemoembolization. Complications associated with embolization and chemoembolization are uncommon; however, several are possible. When an embolic agent travels to an undesired location, it is called a "nontarget" embolization, and the effects that occur are dependent on the organ that has been embolized. "Embolization syndrome," which is a well-described phenomenon in humans, is still being characterized in veterinary patients but likely often includes signs such as lethargy, anorexia, vomiting, and diarrhea. Other potential complications may include organ abscessation, incisional complications, and bleeding.

Whenever possible, resection of liver masses should be pursued, because the outcomes with surgery are excellent.[7] Many liver masses are considered "massive," and resection of one or multiple liver lobes allows for successful control of disease.[7] However, a subset of liver masses occur in challenging locations (eg, right-sided or surrounding major vasculature), and surgical removal may represent significant challenges or be associated with increased morbidity. In these situations, embolization or chemoembolization can be considered if there is an adequate arterial blood supply to the mass. The concept of embolization has been most studied in the liver due to the unique blood supply of the liver and tumors of the liver; most of the tumoral blood supply is arterial, whereas the opposite is true for the blood supply to the normal liver parenchyma.[8] In the veterinary literature, 4 cases of transarterial embolization of canine liver tumors have been described (**Fig. 2**).[9,10]

As tumors often stimulate neovascularization, tumors that are in locations that do not have blood supplies similar to the liver can also be targeted with embolization, as long as blood supply to healthy organs is preserved. Embolization of a cervical/uterine mass in a goat[10] and nasal adenocarcinoma in a cat have been described in the literature.[11] Recently, prostatic embolization was reported[12] and nasal embolization is pursued regularly in the author's practice for the treatment of canine nasal neoplasia.

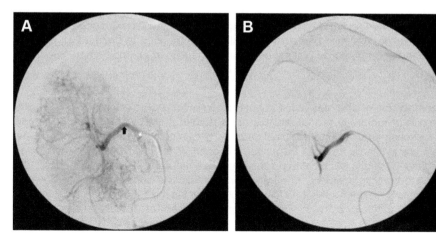

Fig. 2. Embolization of a liver tumor. (*A*) Preembolization: a diagnostic catheter (*asterisk*) has been placed in a hepatic arterial branch (*arrow*), and after injection of contrast medium, opacification of liver tumoral vessels are noted. (*B*) Postembolization: after embolization, tumor opacification is not occurring during injection of contrast medium.

Ablative therapies are generally categorized into chemical and thermal techniques. Most of the clinical data for chemical ablation is focused on the use of ethanol. For this technique, the tumor is identified with ultrasound, and a needle is guided into the tumor. The ethanol is injected directly into the tumor to cause necrosis of tumor cells. Most of the evaluation of ethanol ablation in companion animals has been focused on nonneoplastic disease, such as for the treatment of primary hyperparathyroidism.

Thermal ablation is rarely used for the treatment of nonresectable neoplasia, but instead is chosen for smaller tumors that can often be reached percutaneously or with endoscopic assistance. Currently, ablative therapies are likely the least used IO techniques in companion animals, which can at least partially be explained by a few reasons. Thermal ablation requires expensive equipment and extensive training. The probes that are used during procedures such as radiofrequency ablation and microwave ablation tend to be costly, prohibiting regular use of these devices. In addition, it is unusual for dogs and cats to be diagnosed with tumors of appropriate size (ie, amenable to thermal ablation). For instance, most primary liver or lung tumors in dogs and cats are diagnosed when they are larger in size; however, thermal ablation is regularly used for small tumors in these locations in humans.

DRAINAGE

Interventional techniques are often used for the placement of temporary and permanent drainage catheters. Drains can be placed in luminal organs such as the gallbladder or urinary bladder if obstruction of the outflow of these organs occurs. Cholecystostomy and cystostomy tubes are likely not a good long-term management option for these scenarios due to concerns for infection and dislodgement, but these tubes can be considered for patient stabilization before a more definitive therapy such as surgery or stenting.

The placement of these drainage tubes is generally best accomplished with a combination of ultrasound- and fluoroscopic-guidance. A needle or over-the-needle catheter is introduced into the lumen, and a guide wire is passed through the needle or catheter to maintain access. After removal of the needle or catheter, a multifenestrated tube can be introduced over the guide wire into the lumen and left in place. Locking loop drainage tubes have added protection against accidental removal due to the nature of a suture-locking device that keeps the end of the tubing closed in a coil or "pigtail" shape. A similar placement technique can be used to drain effusions in the thorax and abdomen or to place a catheter for infusion of chemotherapy.

STENTING

Tumor location or size may result in obstruction of luminal structures. When surgical resection of tumors in this situation is not possible or not elected, stent placement can be considered to restore luminal patency. Stents of many shapes, sizes, and materials are available and can be placed via open or minimally invasive techniques. Whenever possible, it is ideal to place stents via a natural orifice to limit the morbidity associated with placement. In companion animals, incisionless minimally invasive techniques have been described for stent placement in the esophagus, colon, urethra, and trachea.[13–20] In addition, image-guided placement of vascular stents has also been reported.[21]

The resection of lower urinary tract neoplasia is often not pursued due to concerns for complications and recurrence. Because many cases of lower urinary tract neoplasia are euthanized or die from local extension and luminal obstruction as opposed to metastatic disease, the treatment of luminal obstruction to allow for expulsion of urine is commonly performed. Treatments such as permanent cystostomy tubes and urinary catheters can be considered but may result in challenging management situations. Urethral stents can be placed easily, with image-guidance and in most cases, provide immediate relief of obstruction.[17–19] In dogs and female cats, placement of urethral stents can be performed through the urethra; in male cats, a small surgical approach with placement in an antegrade fashion is necessary (unless a previous perineal urethrostomy has been performed) due to the size of the delivery system of the urethral stent relative to urethral diameter. For more discussion regarding urethral stenting, see Matthew W. Beal's article, "Interventional Management of Urethral Obstructions, in this issue.

Surgical resection of colonic, esophageal, and tracheal tumors is the treatment of choice for tumors affecting these organs. With extensive luminal obstruction or large tumor burden, removal is not always possible, and stenting can be considered to allow for patency. Stents in this scenario are placed permanently and ramifications should be considered. For stents in the gastrointestinal tract, alterations to the patient's diet may be necessary; regardless, obstruction can still occur.[15] Long-term outcome with the stenting of these cases has been rarely reported,[13–16] but early results in veterinary cases and clinical successes in human patients mandate further evaluation of these techniques.

Vascular stents can be placed to palliate obstructions from large tumors or complications associated with previous surgeries. Vascular obstruction of veins is more likely to occur, and descriptions of vascular stenting in veterinary cases have been limited to hepatic vein and vena cava obstruction.[21] In one case series of 3 dogs with Budd-Chiari syndrome, vascular patency was reestablished after image-guided stent placement.[21]

REFERENCES

1. Bent CL, Low D, Matson MB, et al. Portal vein embolization using a nitinol plug (Amplatzer vascular plug) in combination with histoacryl glue and iodinized oil: adequate hypertrophy with a reduced risk of nontarget embolization. Cardiovasc Intervent Radiol 2009;32:471–7.

2. Kim GC, Bae JH, Ryeom HK. Percutaneous preoperative portal vein embolization using a combination of gelatin sponge and histoacryl glue. Acta Radiol 2009;50:1119–25.

3. Poon R, Fan S, Tsang F, et al. Locoregional therapies for hepatocellular carcinoma: a critical review from the surgeon's perspective. Ann Surg 2002;235:466–86.

4. Culp WT, Mayhew PD, Pascoe PJ, et al. Angiographic anatomy of the major abdominal arterial blood supply in the dog. Vet Radiol Ultrasound 2015;56:474–85.

5. Furness S, Glenny AM, Worthington HV, et al. Interventions for the treatment of oral cavity and oropharyngeal cancer: chemotherapy. Cochrane Database Syst Rev 2010;(9):CD006386.

6. Culp WT, Weisse C, Berent AC, et al. Early tumor response to intraarterial or intravenous administration of carboplatin to treat naturally occurring lower urinary tract carcinoma in dogs. J Vet Intern Med 2015;29:900–7.

7. Liptak JM, Dernell WS, Monnet E, et al. Massive hepatocellular carcinoma in dogs: 48 cases (1992-2002). J Am Vet Med Assoc 2004;225:1225–30.

8. Breedis C, Young G. The blood supply of neoplasms in the liver. Am J Pathol 1954;30:969–77.

9. Cave TA, Johnson V, Beths T, et al. Treatment of unresectable hepatocellular adenoma in dogs with transarterial iodized oil and chemotherapy with and without an embolic agent: a report of two cases. Vet Comp Oncol 2003;1:191–9.

10. Weisse C, Clifford CA, Holt D, et al. Percutaneous arterial embolization and chemoembolization for treatment of benign and malignant tumors in three dogs and a goat. J Am Vet Med Assoc 2002;221:1430–6.

11. Marioni-Henry K, Schwarz T, Weisse C, et al. Cystic nasal adenocarcinoma in a cat treated with piroxicam and chemoembolization. J Am Anim Hosp Assoc 2007;43:347–51.

12. Culp WTN, Johnson EG, Palm CA, et al. Prostatic artery embolization: early results of a novel treatment for prostatic neoplasia in canine patients, in Proceedings. Veterinary Society of Surgical Oncology Meeting, Napa (CA), 2016.

13. Hansen KS, Weisse C, Berent AC, et al. Use of a self-expanding metallic stent to palliate esophageal neoplastic obstruction in a dog. J Am Vet Med Assoc 2012; 240:1202–7.

14. Hume DZ, Solomon JA, Weisse CW. Palliative use of a stent for colonic obstruction caused by adenocarcinoma in two cats. J Am Vet Med Assoc 2006;228: 392–6.

15. Culp WT, MacPhail CM, Perry JA, et al. Use of a nitinol stent to palliate a colorectal neoplastic obstruction in a dog. J Am Vet Med Assoc 2011;239:222–7.

16. Culp WT, Weisse C, Cole SG, et al. Intraluminal tracheal stenting for treatment of tracheal narrowing in three cats. Vet Surg 2007;36:107–13.

17. Blackburn AL, Berent AC, Weisse CW, et al. Evaluation of outcome following urethral stent placement for the treatment of obstructive carcinoma of the urethra in dogs: 42 cases (2004-2008). J Am Vet Med Assoc 2013;242:59–68.

18. McMillan SK, Knapp DW, Ramos-Vara JA, et al. Outcome of urethral stent placement for management of urethral obstruction secondary to transitional cell carcinoma in dogs: 19 cases (2007-2010). J Am Vet Med Assoc 2012;241:1627–32.

19. Weisse C, Berent A, Todd K, et al. Evaluation of palliative stenting for management of malignant urethral obstructions in dogs. J Am Vet Med Assoc 2006; 229:226–34.

20. Brace MA, Weisse C, Berent A. Preliminary experience with stenting for management of non-urolith urethral obstruction in eight cats. Vet Surg 2014;43:199–208.

21. Schlicksup MD, Weisse CW, Berent AC, et al. Use of endovascular stents in three dogs with Budd-Chiari syndrome. J Am Vet Med Assoc 2009;235:544–50.

Moving?

Make sure your subscription moves with you!

To notify us of your new address, find your **Clinics Account Number** (located on your mailing label above your name), and contact customer service at:

Email: journalscustomerservice-usa@elsevier.com

800-654-2452 (subscribers in the U.S. & Canada)
314-447-8871 (subscribers outside of the U.S. & Canada)

Fax number: 314-447-8029

Elsevier Health Sciences Division
Subscription Customer Service
3251 Riverport Lane
Maryland Heights, MO 63043

*To ensure uninterrupted delivery of your subscription, please notify us at least 4 weeks in advance of move.

Printed and bound by CPI Group (UK) Ltd, Croydon, CR0 4YY

03/10/2024

01040388-0013